HOW TO LOSE YOUR VIRGINITY
(...and how not to)

by Shawn Wickens

INTRODUCTION	2 – 7
1. YOU'LL NEVER BELIEVE WHAT HAPPENED TO ME	8 – 21
2. HOW DO YOU PUT THESE THINGS ON?	22 – 29
3. PENIS IS THE PROPER WORD. VULVA IS THE PROPER WORD	30 – 45
4. IT'S NOT THAT BAD. IF IT WAS, EVERYONE WOULDN'T BE DOING IT	46 – 55
5. WHAT'S GOING ON IN THERE?	56 – 67
6. TONIGHT IS THE NIGHT YOU MAKE ME A WOMAN / MAN	68 – 81
7. JUST FELL INTO IT	82 – 93
8. I HAVE TWO RUBBERS. WEAR THEM BOTH, IT WILL DESENSITIZE YOU	94 – 107
9. WE DROP KICKED OUR CHERRIES	108 – 119
10. IT WAS A TRAIN WRECK	120 – 139
11. MEN CAN BE SUCH PIGS	140 – 149
12. NO MEANS NO	150 – 165
13. THAT'S ME IN THE SPOTLIGHT, LOSING MY RELIGION	166 – 179
14. IF I HAD THE CHANCE 2 DO IT ALL AGAIN I WOULDN'T CHANGE A STROKE…	180 – 203
15. GOING TO THE CHAPEL AND WE'RE GOING TO GET MARRIED	204 – 207
16. I NEVER DID IT!	208 – 213
17. THE OTHER SIDE: TAKING VIRGINITY	214 – 223
18. I DID IT MY WAY	224 – 233
CONCLUSION	234
SPECIAL THANKS	235

© Shawn Wickens

INTRODUCTION

Origin of the Project

Through a friend, I received a handful of free passes to the 27th annual Cleveland International Film Festival. One of the many features I watched that year was a German film *Mein Bruder, der Vampir* (2001), the story of a girl's quest to find the best person with whom to lose her virginity. We see her several unsuccessful attempts with numerous inadequate suitors and I'll wait until the next section to spoil the ending, but I left the theater thinking, "If this story exists, what else is out there?"

Later that night I went to a festival after-party and my thoughts dwelled on both my first sexual experience and that of the character from the film. Whenever the subject of sex came up among friends, talking about virginity was always taboo. I realized that I knew very few of their stories, and of those who did venture to share, the experience was always blown off as "awkward."

On a whim, and fueled by the courage of an open bar, I asked some fellow festival-goers what they thought of the film with the intent of steering the conversation toward their own loss of virginity story. I was surprised how open and receptive people were to such a personal and private inquiry from a stranger. Even more so, I was surprised to find out how entertaining and intriguing I found everyone's responses. The amateur ethnographer in me had awoken.

Intent

Personally, I had mixed feelings about my own first time. I was excited when it happened, pleased who it happened with. But the girl was more experienced than I, so I never told her it was my first time and I always regretted that I wasn't more honest and open about the moment. Over time, that was what I focused on whenever I thought back on it.

Prior to my own first, I would hear other people talking about their first time and how awkward it was, so that's what I came to expect. And certainly, compared to subsequent and more experienced times, they *are* awkward or clumsy. I started thinking that perhaps we are not only taught to expect nothing less than awkward, but in some cases, over time, we tend to forget the relief, joy, and triumph of the first sexual experience and remember simply the awkwardness. I heard the term "awkward" thrown around so much that perhaps it started to eclipse the other feelings I had.

One of the concepts from my college psychology courses that fascinated me the most was the idea of learned helplessness; the notion that presented with a constant and negative stimulus, we learn to accept or feel that we have no control over the situation. The example used in class was administering electrical shocks over a period of time to caged lab mice. When their cages were left open, the mice made no attempt at escape because they perceived their situation to be hopeless.

The story in *Mein Bruder, der Vampir* although fictional, presented an extreme alternative, a unique story. In it, the main character, Nicole, decides the best person to have sex with is someone she trusts. That person ends up being her developmentally disabled, older brother because as she sees it, this will also be an opportunity to give him something. Different, disturbing, but not awkward – that is how she chose to do it. And this triggered in my mind that all first times can't be horrible; they certainly can't all be great, either. There has to be a range of emotions, consequences,

I then set out to dispel the myth, or at least the pre-conceived notion, that all first times are lame. Inspired by the story from *Mein Bruder, der Vampir*, I knew that there existed out in the world a whole spectrum of loss of virginity stories. And if this were true, I would set out and find them.

Why a Book?

At the time I was working at a public access cable TV station in Amherst, Ohio as well as doing freelance video production jobs in my hometown of Cleveland. As this was the medium I had access to, my initial thought was a documentary. However, it but being the summer of 2003, "Girls Gone Wild" infomercials were all over late-night TV. And as a direct reaction to the popularity of those videos, I wanted the project to have more of a journalistic and sincere inquiry into the stories than a raucous, hedonistic, in-your-face portrayal of sexuality. And with a camera present, raucous and vulgar is what I thought the footage would spiral towards.

I wanted honesty and openness and I figured a small tape recorder would capture that more easily than an obtrusive camera. A collection of these interviews in book format seemed to me a more civilized approach.

Methodology

On my first evening out with the tape recorder, I didn't intend to interview anyone. I planned on only testing the microphone and its functionality under noisy background conditions. I met up with my friend Anne Marie Kozlowski at a bar and she asked what the tape recorder was for. I said, "To test it." "To test it for what?" "To see how well it works." I was avoiding the subject. "OK, but what for?" I acquiesced and she found the idea fascinating and forced me to commit her story to audio tape. Other friends and friends of friends found out what I was doing and wanted to share their experiences as well. Thirteen stories later, my tape recorder test was more successful than expected.

Many of my subsequent interviews were recorded in bars because it felt like the appropriate setting to breach the subject of sex. I took great care in not approaching anyone who was too inebriated to make an informed decision on sharing their story. Also, all interviewees signed a release form acknowledging that their contribution was for a book. Everyone was informed that theirs and any other names they mentioned would be changed.

Other locations I interviewed people included coffee houses, house parties, galleries, political rallies, concerts – anywhere people congregated. I had experimented with randomly stopping people on the street but quickly learned that this approach was a little too unsettling for them and me.

Over time, and after some nervous first attempts, I settled into my quick and concise introduction: "Hi. My name is Shawn Wickens. I'm currently traveling the country, working on a book about loss of virginity stories. Do you have a story you'd like to share?"

A thousand people seemed like a nice, round number to shoot for and certainly enough to give me a wide range of interesting, humorous, poignant stories, and even tragic ones.

In order to cast as wide a net as possible, I visited the following cities on several road trips over a three-year period.

On a few occasions, I coordinated road trips to certain cities during events that would draw a lot of people: the 2004 Democratic and Republican National Conventions in Boston and New York, George Bush's second inauguration in Washington D.C., Mardi Gras in New Orleans. The full list of cities includes:

- **New York, NY**
- **Los Angeles, CA**
- **San Francisco, CA**
- **Chicago, IL**
- **Boston, MA**
- **Denver, CO**
- **Washington D.C.**
- **Philadelphia, PA**
- **Cleveland, OH**
- **New Orleans, LA**
- **Austin, TX**
- **Mobile, AL**
- **Providence, RI**
- **Hoboken, NJ**
- **Greensboro, NC**
- **Louisville, KY**
- **Nashville, TN**
- **Memphis, TN**
- **Tulsa, OK**
- **Amarillo, TX**
- **Burlington, VA**
- **Savannah, GA**
- **Port Charlotte, FL**
- **Gainesville, FL**
- **Roswell, NM**
- **Tucson, AZ**
- **Phoenix, AZ**
- **Reno, NV**
- **Salt Lake City, UT**
- **Colorado Springs, CO**
- **Wichita, KS**
- **Des Moines, IA**
- **Raleigh, NC**
- **Gettysburg, PA**
- **Montreal, QC CANADA**

I then transcribed these interviews, and the full text of some appear in the book. The rest, I edited down for conciseness, taking care to include all of the relevant information and keep the speaker's voice intact.

Presentation

Chapters are arranged by overall mood of the story (ranging from good to bad) in addition to stories that have a religious influence, the process of buying, acquiring, or when putting on a condom played a role, etc. Throughout the book I've included facts on sexuality and virginity as well as quotes that I found relevant, interesting or simply random (along with a fake name, age at the time of the interview, location of experience). These come from stories that didn't make the final draft.

Although I was originally interested in stories that reflected a positive memory, I also include in this collection a few of the stories that reflect the less successful sexual experiences, as well as some of the negative ones because as much could be learned from the bad as well as the good.

I don't purport to revealing the definite and absolute best way to lose one's virginity.
There's no perfect method to ensure a good first time. There's no road map, no checklist of enumerated steps of exactly what needs to happen when. What works for some people doesn't work for others. The hope is, other than the entertainment value, that through exploring these stories, it will compel those on the verge of their sexual lives to put more thought into what they want and need out of their first time – to make an informed decision. It is my hope that this book will allow the rest of us to reflect on our first experiences and cherish them – or put them behind us.

Limitations

Much to the dismay, I'd gather, of my former college professors (undergrad and graduate), this is hardly a scientific study but more of a snapshot or overview of the people I randomly spoke with during my travels. Early on I decided against collecting demographic information as I feared people would balk about revealing personal details and intimate stories, as well as discussing income, ethnicity and occupation. Thus each story includes merely a pseudonym and their age at the time of the interview.

It was difficult to separate some of the stories into chapters. There is a flood of emotions associated with the first time. So much grey area exists in relation to these stories that I often had to arbitrarily choose the overriding theme in which the story fit. For example, getting caught in the act doesn't presuppose the quality of the act. Some of those who were caught were horrified; for others, it didn't negatively affect the moment.

Given the locations I frequented, the age range of subjects is skewed younger than I would've liked. That had as much to do with the higher percentage of older people who turned down interview requests, many noting that they couldn't remember or (and I think this answer is closer to the truth) were less open about the topic as opposed to younger generations.

My story - I'll call her Alice.

In fairness to those reading and to all who anonymously shared their experiences, I will openly share mine.

I was a little older than many of the contributors to this book. Because of several circumstances – a religious background, going to an all-boys high school, apprehension at getting a girl pregnant, pride, a long-distance relationship in college, learned helplessness (simply getting used to not going all the way) – I waited until shortly after my 22nd birthday.

I started dating a girl shortly after I transferred to a different college and quickly discovered that she was more experienced than I was. For fear of being judged harshly or seen as being inferior, I kept my history vague.

I was past the legal drinking age, some of my fellow and fellow late-bloomers were starting to "drop" and I began feeling that I had held on to my v-card a little too long. I was casually seeing a woman who didn't share in my hang-ups, so I could sense that my time was fast approaching.

When it came time for the conversation, Alice said that she wanted to wait, that in the past she had rushed into physical relationships and that she liked me and just wanted to wait, which was fine with me. I wasn't about to dive headfirst into an area that I only had minimal experience.

We were at her house late one night, her mother was sequestered for jury duty on a highly publicized murder trial. We were in her bed, not watching the television, and making out as we always did when we had the chance. I don't know where I came up with this line; at the time I thought it was quite inspired but since then, looking back, I laugh about it. I said to her, "How about we take off our clothes and just lay here." Alice laughed, we each disrobed under the blankets and she reached to the side table and grabbed a condom.

My line had elicited the results I deep down had hoped for but I was severely unprepared for what my next course of action was. My first attempt at putting on the condom was a bust and she pointed out that I was putting it on backwards. I casually commented that I would just put it on the other way but she expertly pointed out that it was already "used." So she got another one and took charge putting it on while I assisted.

"How could she not know?" I thought. "She has to at least suspect." Or maybe she chalked up my nervousness as excitement. Sex is exciting and I'm guessing that she was excited too. So maybe she didn't think much about how un-adept I was leading up to it.

She then took it upon herself to make sure everything "fit properly" and smoothly. One less thing for me to think about.

Now, I wasn't a complete amateur. I had had other experiences so I had some slight confidence in my stamina and my ability to perform. I remember the phrase "This is happening. This is happening," running over and over through my head. And something along the lines of, "Right now, I'm having sex," also came up.

And I really was into the girl, I was attracted to her, I liked her, so the elation of not only doing the act but who I was doing it with kept entering my brain. Concentrating on all of that took some of the pressure off of wanting to do it well.

When the twin bed we were on began to make too much noise, for concern of waking up her younger sister in the next room, she suggested we move to the floor. It was there that I "finished" but wanting to really give a stellar time my first try out of the gates, I kept going. When fatigue finally set in just minutes later, I faked having an orgasm so I could stop and rest.

I don't recall specifics of the post-sex conversation, but if she thought I was an amateur, she didn't let on.

The next morning I drove home and felt a mix of disbelief, excitement, and euphoria. I wanted to high five everybody, not to boast but to celebrate. I felt really good about myself. There existed no thoughts of lameness. If anything, I felt like a winner. And despite our efforts to conceal what we shared, her older sister had seen my car in the driveway when she left for work and once jury duty was over, shared with their mother that, "Shawn spent the night," wink-wink. I would later find out that my staying over was revealed at the dinner table, so no repercussions there. No problem.

Over time I got better, more adept. My rookie status, as it were, was never called into question. And I just grew accustomed to not telling her that she took my virginity.

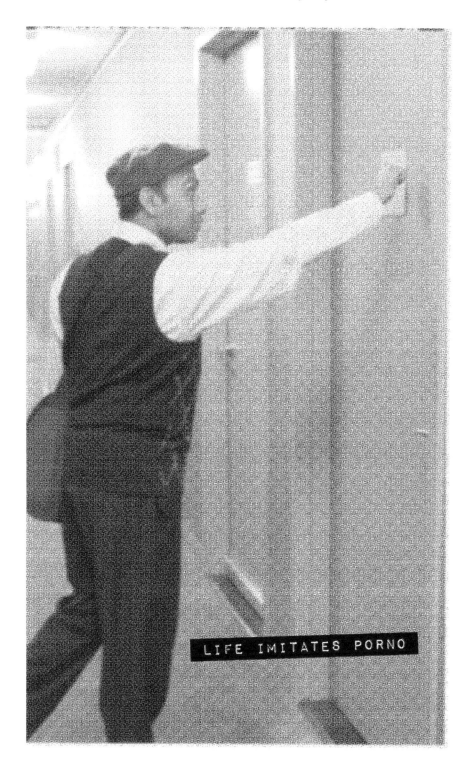

(...and how not to)

"YOU'LL NEVER BELIEVE WHAT HAPPENED TO ME."

1

When I met Vivian, I was speaking to a group of ladies out in the Warehouse District of Cleveland, Ohio for a bachelorette party. The bride-to-be was visibly shocked when she heard one of her bridesmaids tell of her evening of sex with a married man.

The title for "MY PARENTS PROBABLY WOULDN'T EVEN BELIEVE ME IF I TOLD THEM WHERE I WAS" was inspired by an actual quote from Zoe, an 18-year-old I met in Nashville. She was hanging out at a coffee house on a Saturday night because, as she put it, her wild times were behind her.

After I spoke with Shigeru I found myself asking him if it really happened. He assured me it had, he seemed very genuine, and his story was even verified by his then-girlfriend who had heard it before. So, it's so crazy, it must be true! Right?

Teachers, threesomes, porn stars... it really happens.

WE WERE ONLY FRESHMEN
Barry, 28

This began when I was 14 years old, the summer going into my freshman year in Catholic high school. I had had my first kiss only three weeks earlier. It was also the same time I started drinking and partying. Kind of young for that kind of stuff but I'm from Iowa where 14 is about the average. It's Fourth of July weekend and I'm at this party flirting with a real cute girl, same age as me, who's already dating a senior: Dolph.

She was a big fan of blackberry brandy but couldn't hold it, couldn't handle herself. Everyone knew she was the type of girl who got drunk and liked to mess around. She was drunk, I was drunk, and we snuck into the guy's room who was throwing the party.

Her boyfriend, the senior, happened to be a middle linebacker for our varsity football team. I was already warned. I was warned when I was flirting with her. Her boyfriend was one of those guys who would go up to people and say, "Head or gut?" And if you said gut, he'd punch you in the head. If you said head, you know, vice-versa. So I knew what I was getting myself into. Nevertheless, I'm 14, and this is about to be the first time I ever showed my penis to a woman. I was really insecure about it because I was a 150-lb drunk pothead. You know, how could I physically compete against a 270-lb middle linebacker. But we had beautiful sex, listening to "The End" by The Doors and we were both big Doors fans. She said it was great.

The linebacker found out, everybody found out. So once school starts, big ol' Dolph sees me on the bridge and I just about shit my pants. He throws down his books, holds up a fist and asks me, "Head or gut?" I was like, "Dude. I'm really sorry. I didn't know. I didn't know." He spit chewing tobacco all over my books. That was the worst of it. The way I looked at it, this 270-lb senior got hosed by a freshman. He was a football player, I was a nobody and I had a great time humping on his girlfriend.

It turned out that my best friend all through high school, who I hadn't met at that point, he was the guy whose bed I lost my virginity in. And he and the girl I lost my virginity to ended up getting married three years ago. That took place when I was 14, I'm 26 now and I was the best man at their wedding. I'm not sure if Nate knows and he's like a brother to me. I'm sure she hasn't mentioned it to him. But the fact that it was in his bedroom, I'm now his best friend, and was the best man at their wedding, I think makes it a good story. Everyone I tell seems to like it... except for Nate, who I've never told.

> You'd be amazed what two naked people can do in a movie theater. It was a long movie. It was a hell of an experience doing it during and not really watching, *As Good as It Gets*. I own two copies of it on DVD for memory's sake. One is still wrapped in the plastic for posterity.
>
> *Jake, 24*
> *Ocala, Florida*

(...and how not to)

DÉJÀ VU
Maddie, 21

I was with my boyfriend at a party at one of our friends' houses. We were doing this camping thing-a-majing, there was a bonfire and everyone had blankets on the ground, We were making out and he climbed on top of me and said, "Can I?" and you know, I was drunk. We decided to have sex right then and there.

I thought it was gonna be a big deal, but afterwards I was like, "That's it?" I mean it is a big deal when you're young, you don't even know the emotional effects it has on you. I think sex put a strain on the relationship that, as kids, we weren't ready for.

So I went home with one of my friends, she was actually at the party with me. I told her that I slept with my boyfriend and she was like, "Well have you ever slept with a girl?" And I said, "No." So she slept over and we slept with each other.

It was a better experience with her. It was more sensual, more erotic I guess. Maybe more crazy and daring. Maybe that's what made it better.

But my brother found out and told everybody. That was harsh. My parents found out and that wasn't good either. Now they're more supportive about my sexuality. My mom still has issues but my dad is happy as long as I'm happy.

About a year ago, I get home from my college and my parents tell me that they're moving and they bought a house. They tell me the address and it turns out to be the house where I lost my virginity with the guy in the backyard. That's the house they're in now. My dad laughed but my mom just rolled her eyes. She wishes I was still with guys.

SO... WHAT BRINGS YOU HERE?
Jimmy, 43

I was living in London, lived there from when I was 10 to 19. I lost mine to a Scottish junkie in a squat in World's End, this section of London. Iggy Pop's album, *The Idiot* was playing... the song "Tiny Girls." I was dealing at the time, so I guess you could say she was a customer of mine.

This girl, she had just broken up with her boyfriend. She was pissed off and wanted to screw somebody to get back at her boyfriend and I was happy to step up. It was just fate, "Yeah, why not." I was 14 so she was, well... an older woman. She was like 18.

The thing that was weird about it was the next morning I went down to the kitchen to get some stale corn flakes and this other girl I went to school with was there. She had lost her virginity the same night to a male junkie in the same freaking squat. We were both too cool to acknowledge anything that happened so we just sat down and looked at each other and ate breakfast. I ended up dating her. Yeah, so it was very bizarre and pleasant.

Then two weeks later they tore down the squat. So all I have left is the album – Iggy Pop.

PB & J
Mario, 30

I discovered sex when a fellow male classmate and I had sex on my parents' kitchen table. We were 14, we were there, it happened, and we needed lube. We could be so lucky to have butter or olive oil. All I could find was crunchy peanut butter. It served its purpose. When we were done I cleaned the kitchen table with a mop. I was real paranoid about it because I had to sit at the kitchen table and have breakfast with my family the next morning. They suspected nothing but could probably tell I was a little bit happier than usual.

> I broke into the storeroom where the cameras were monitored and stole the videotape so I got myself losing my virginity on tape. I know how long it was, the exact date, the exact time… everything.
>
> *Calvin, 22*
> *Carmel, Indiana*

HAPPY BIRTHDAY… MR. PRESIDENT
Seth, 24

To tell you the truth I don't really remember her name. I want to say it was Raquel or Rochelle, something like that. When I turned 16 my dad decided that I was getting to that age where I was old enough to meet girls and stuff so for my birthday party he gets me a chick who pops out of this huge ass birthday cake. It was totally unexpected. I just thought he had this huge birthday cake decoration. Everyone thought that, and then a woman jumps out of it.

It was a PG affair, she wasn't topless but later on I got to see them anyway. It was a pretty big bash, family and friends were there. My stepmom flipped out because this girl was like an escort. She was pretty hot, I got to talking to her and she was sitting on my lap pretty much the entire party. It was pretty fun, you know having an attractive lady show me all that attention who, granted was getting paid to be there – jump out of the cake and surprise me, but one thing led to another.

She asked me, "Do you want to come to my place later?" I was like, "Hell yeah!" I was 16-years-old, I had a sexual libido from hell. You know at that age when it kicks in all you need is a hole with a heartbeat, let alone a sexy escort.

After the party I told my folks I was going over my friend Tony's to hang out and chill with some buddies. I got in her car, went to her place and she pretty much told me what to do. Showed me what it's like to have sex and stuff. Then I rode home on my skateboard.

(...and how not to)

LIFE IMITATES PORNO
Shigeru N, 25

SHIGERU N: I used to deliver newspapers. In Japan. This was an area that had a real tight community, a bunch of tall buildings and whatnot. So one day... I delivered newspapers and at the same time I collected for the bill.

SHAWN WICKENS: How old were you?

SN: I was... I think I was 14, if not 15. Around that age. At this one apartment that I delivered newspapers to, the owner was a porn star. She asked me to come in and we talked and she asked me a bunch of shit about my sexual experience and I told her I had none. She asked if I was interested or not, and of course her being gorgeous and an older woman.

SW: Was she a porn star that you were familiar with?

SN: No, not really. But later that day I told some people at work that and they were familiar with her. They recognized that she was living in this particular apartment building. But she basically seduced me and led me to the loss-of-virginity experience.

SW: Did you continue going there for awhile?

SN: No, no, no. Actually that's a funny thing because I was so scared. At the same time people made fun of me, that was the talk of the company, the talk of the town. And I don't really like the attention so I stopped going. I asked my boss if I could change my route to a different place. And... so that never happened again but supposedly she had called a couple times asking for me. So... that's it. It was weird.

SW: Are you aware of her doing that with anybody else?

SN: You know what, I asked her if she had done this before or not, and she said, "No." But she had this smile that made me think she possibly had.

SW: Afterwards did you see any of her movies?

SN: Yes I did. Yes I did. And she looked nothing like she did when I had seen her personally. Like the level of intensity was completely different. When I was with her she was very teacher-like instead of being really... a slob. I saw her on video once. And that's it, and I never went back.
    I remember that it wasn't that good. I was excited and I was as hard as I could get. But I actually... the whole experience wasn't as exciting as I wanted it to be. I asked her... if mine was big or not. Decent size? And she said, "Yes." That boosted my confidence in a way.

SW: Did you remember to collect money?

SN: Yes I did collect money. Yes I did. She was very nice.

MY PARENTS PROBABLY WOULDN'T EVEN BELIEVE ME IF I TOLD THEM WHERE I WAS
Zoe, 18

I was 13, at an Applebee's with a friend. Our waiter was this guy Troy and I asked him to take me back to the freezer, stick a chicken nugget in my mouth, put my legs behind my head, and fuck me. And he did it. I don't know how I came up with that. I was a little messed up on drugs, high on ecstasy and weed. I used to be a little crazy but I've grown up since then. My friend just sat in the booth by herself cracking up about it. It is pretty funny if you think about it. I can't remember how long it lasted, but I was late for curfew that night.

I've settled down since then.

BACK OF THE BUS
Caitlin, 39

It was with my school bus driver. His name was Frank. He was hot. I had been flirting with him probably since I was about 13-years-old. He never knew I was a virgin but I played it off like I was a little slut.

So he came over my parents' house. Our house people were gone and he brought a friend over. I thought the friend was going to sit downstairs but he was really attractive and I have a thing for black men so we all ended up going upstairs to my mother's room.

I didn't look my age back then. I could get into bars. I looked older so I think it made me act a little older. Frank was maybe about 24.

We stayed up in that room for hours. It was the perfect setting for a first fuck. It was the first time I had ever given head. The best thing was that I'd never thought about receiving oral sex, but it happened and I loved it. First time I had ever had sex and I ended up fucking two men at the same time. It was probably the hottest sexual experience I'd ever had. We started and it went on and on and on. The housekeeper came in the next morning. I guess she straightened up after we left and she never said anything about it to my mother.

> We did all the things every couple does at prom... went to the dance, had some drinks and stuff. And then we decided, you know, already lost the virginity the night before... we might as well just have anal on prom night to still make it a special night.
> I think she was the one who brought it up and since we had messed it up kind of the night before; she felt like she deserved to give something else up the next night. It was good.
>
> *Jay, 21*
> *Tacoma, Washington*

(...and how not to)

TAKING WORK HOME WITH YOU
Dylan, 36

I truly, truly lost my virginity at the age of 12. I used to cut grass for spending money and I cut my sixth-grade math teacher's grass. I happened to go in for some lemonade and she's sitting in a T-shirt and panties grading papers. We get into a conversation and she asks me about some of the students. The teacher kind of looks like Diana Ross, very beautiful. She started to ask about which kids had a crush on her, who had a crush on other students, that sort of talk. Then she asked me if I ever French kissed, and if I knew what that was. I said, "No." So she showed me how to French kiss. Then she asked me if I ever had any sex with a woman. Again I told her, "No." So she showed me that too. Wound up having sex with my sixth-grade math teacher right there on her living room floor.

She didn't have to tell me not to tell anybody. It was just the one time but she showed me more things than I thought possible. It was like I was thrown into a whole new category. The girls my age may have thought I was immature but that gave me a little reference point that I wasn't as immature as they thought.

I got my normal $15 fee, some lemonade, and a little extra credit. And it turned me into the person that I am today: a womanizer, a love for the older women.

MULTIPLE FELONIES
Roger, 27

This involves a stolen vehicle, the Internet, and her mom sleeping on the couch next to us. It started out with me stealing a credit card and getting a fake AOL account. I then met this girl over the Internet who lived a few miles away. We were talking online for about a week on some AOL chat room. One night she dared me to come out and see her, bet me I wouldn't do it. I was like, "I guarantee you. I'll even bet you 50 bucks that I'll be there in half an hour.

This was before I had a car, didn't even have a license yet. So I stole the neighbor's car, found a key under the visor, worst place to leave one. I show up at her doorstop and the look on her face was, "Holy shit I actually owe this guy 50 bucks." I meet her mom. We hang out for a couple hours watching TV waiting for her mom to fall asleep. But she fell asleep on the couch so we did it on the floor with her mom asleep right there.

She gave me the worst blowjob of my life and she did actually give me the 50 dollars, babysitting money or something. Turns out, years later I became good friends with her older brother and I found out that at the time the girl was only 13.

I did get caught for the stolen vehicle and the stolen credit card. I was facing 15 years in federal prison for bank fraud but somehow I avoided punishment. I have no idea why but I guess they dropped everything.

TWO GENERATIONS
Simon, 31

All the kids used to ask me, you know because we used to have to shower together, "Why you already got hair on your balls?" and, "Why's your dick so big?" First time I ever had sex was with my friend's mom. My friend's sister blew me and told her mom I had a big dick. So the mom took me in the closet and pulled my pants down. I put my feet up against the door and fucked the shit out of my best friend's mom.

I have no idea how old the mom was but this was the summer between sixth and seventh grade and I was grown enough to bust a nut.

Then I did the sister too.

(also has a story in the chapter "Taking It", see page 220)

NEWSPAPER CLIPPINGS
George, 22

I had a party at my house back when I was in high school. I'm sitting on the couch, having a good time and then all of a sudden this girl was all on my piece. She was a friend of a friend from a different school, next town over. And then some kid came and sat in between us, and my buddy was like, "Hey man, you're cock-blocking." He said, "Oh. Sorry. My bad." I think the kid was wasted. Then, later on that night she was just on my shit again. Next thing I knew... she ripped all my clothes off and we had crazy sex all night. I never called her after, she never called me, never talked to her ever again.

A few months later I was leaving on a trip for Spain for seven months. The day I left the morning newspaper said: "Girl Dies Mysterious Death". It was her, the girl from my party. They were speculating it was like a drug overdose, but the actual cause was a mystery. So... the girl I lost my virginity with died like the day before I left for Spain. It really creeped me out. It was really weird that I never saw her again or *could* never see her again. She was a nice girl but it was just, all right, took my virginity one night, thanks a lot. And then she was dead and I took a plane across the world and kind of started a new chapter of my life. It was a weird fate type of feeling. It creeped me out but it was interesting taking a plane and then showing up somewhere else and it gave me a story to tell when I got there.

But... I don't know, it's also sort of interesting that the person who I lost my virginity to is no longer with us. I can never talk to her about that, can never relate to her about that. You know, so it's just mine, it's only my experience now. No one else can share in it.

Maybe I wonder if I had called her the next day would she be alive. Sure I've thought that, you never know what would have been different. But it was a mysterious death. They never really said. I think she was 17 or 18. Yup. She was hot.

(...and how not to)

THE DIAGNOSIS
Tammy I, 47

SHAWN WICKENS: So tell me about who it was with...

TAMMY I: I was 22 years old. I was told that I had leukemia and I had just come out of a nunnery and I was a virgin.

SHAWN WICKENS: And you found that you had leukemia so then you left the nunnery?

TI: No, no, no. When I was high school age I went through a nunnery. I eventually chose not to do that anymore, realized it wasn't for me and left. I was originally from Minnesota but moved to Texas, got a job, and was put in the hospital for exhaustion and when they ran the tests they said that I had leukemia. So while they're in the process of running other tests I'm thinking to myself, "I am not going to die a virgin. Got to figure this out." So I went out and lived a very precarious life for two months but in the process I found a boyfriend, he was living in Houston and I called him up. I was in East Texas. And I said, "You have to come tonight."

SW: How had you met him?

TI: I met him through work. We were both supervisors for an oil company. So he comes over to the house, I drank a huge gallon of wine, not even the good stuff. We were in the throes of passion and he says to me, "Do you have a condom?" And I was like "What would I have a condom for? I'm a virgin." And he says, "Well... what can we use?" He went out into the kitchen and he comes back with a bread bag, which the crumbs were kind of interesting as far as texture goes. And so that is my virgin story... I lost my virginity with a bread bag.

SW: And I guess it worked.

TI: He was 35, I was 22. I was over it. About a month and a half later they told me I did not have leukemia. I only had mono. The doctor told me the properties were the same. I've found out since then that that is not true.

SW: After you found that out were you upset that you were driven to lose your virginity under false pretenses?

TI: No. No. I had a fellow he used to come into my stores all the time, a black truck driver, a short little guy out of Carthage, Texas. Everyone called him Black Magic and he would tell me that I needed the package. Coming out of a nunnery I had no idea what the package was. When I finally *got* the package it was a revelation for me. Kind of a Catholic revelation story.

I figured out, after the fact that it actually made me live every day for what it's worth. I have no regrets on anything I've ever done, ever said... anything. The sex probably, quite honestly was the best thing that came out of that whole mess.

How to Lose Your Virginity

HOME SCHOOLED
Marius P, 28

MARIUS P: How did I lose my virginity? My mother.

SHAWN WICKENS: Really?

MP: I'm not kidding.

SW: How old were you?

MP: I was eight.

SW: Did you like, know what was going on?

MP: See what happened was... my father sucked so bad in bed that she wasn't about to have her offspring suck in bed.

SW: That's the explanation she gave you?

MP: That was her explanation. Fucked up or not... she taught me how to eat pussy. I'm not kidding you.

SW: How did it happen? Were you just like in bed and...

MP: She's fucked up. She's got major problems in the head. These days they would consider that child abuse. I consider it child abuse. But now, as an adult, I think it's the best goddamn thing she ever taught me. So what can you do?

SW: How did she start it?

MP: I recall her coming home drunk... then she put my hand on the fucking table and played fucking chicken with a knife. That's how it got started. Crazy fucked-up shit. It's a fucked-up way but... you know, what can you say? Shit happens.

(see page 212)

I was losing terribly at Monopoly, very badly. This other girl had Park Place, but I had Boardwalk. So I offered her oral sex for Park Place and two grand in Monopoly money. We went into the bathroom. That's how it began.

Brody, 21
New York, New York

(...and how not to)

THE UNIVERSE WORKS IN MYSTERIOUS WAYS
Taryn, 24

I was 13 and mad at my parents so I ran away from home. I can't even remember what the fight was about. It was really just an excuse to go to my room early so I could sneak out my window and catch a train to meet a guy from a different state.

He was a drug dealer from Florida that I met through friends of friends. He was into the rave scene, listened to the Dead Kennedys and The Chemical Brothers and sold crystal meth, ecstasy, and ketamine. At the time I did nothing harder than weed.

He had a very complicated family situation and he was in Connecticut for the weekend visiting his parents and step parents or something. So my girlfriend and I took the Metro North train from Grand Central up to somewhere in Connecticut. He picked us up and drove us somewhere, all I remember was it was by the water; a one-bedroom studio, a very temporary kind of setup. I'm a gentlewoman and my man was a gentleman so we let his friend and my friend take the bed. The drug dealer and I took the closet.

It was a closet with those sliding doors, so we laid down on the carpet and slid the door shut. Like I said, I was 13 and I had never really done it before. I'm a small person and was even smaller years ago. He was at least five years older and over six feet tall, so he was a weight to bear.

We discussed it briefly beforehand. It was consensual, it was safe. There was a lot of pain and suffering but I got through it with rug burns and it was a beautiful experience. He asked if it hurt. I said, "Yes," and he said, "OK. That's probably normal." I was shocked at how sweet he actually was about it, given my stereotype of drug dealers at the time.

Then this whole weird episode turned unfortunate because my parents managed to track me down to tell me my Great Aunt Gerda had died. She was an amazing woman who moved to the Lower East Side after escaping from Nazi Germany. She settled down with a jeweler, became a jeweler herself. Anyway that's who died the night I lost it. Talk about feeling responsible for something in the cosmic sense. You know, being a self-centered person at the time, I thought I had something to do with it. So I came home.

I was expecting to never hear from the guy again, but he started persistently calling me. The guy got so attached so I swore never to give my number out on a one-night stand again. I never ran away from home again either. I suppose that was less of a conscious decision and more of a lack of need. I got my space from my parents anyway because after that incident they sent me off to boarding school.

GIRLS GONE WILD
Frank, 23

We used to party over at my buddy's place. His parents were straight off the boat from Poland; both PhDs, both very intelligent people. One was a raging alcoholic, the other barely spoke a word of English. The dad would be 16 drinks deep by the time we'd get to the place. He used to drive drunk into town and pick up steak filets and beer for us. Go back to the house and we'd have raging barbecue keggers.

The parents were successful business people. They had a hot tub, which was perfect for us. I guess the parents just didn't give a fuck what we did. The mom would walk around topless in just her underwear. The dad built his own stereo systems and we used to chill out with him and listen to music. I actually got into the Rolling Stones because of him.

This was in high school about the time people started hooking up with each other and everything. Two girls and I, we were hanging out in the hot tub. We were all friends and I had fooled around with one of them before. They were best friends and pretty drunk and we were all in our underwear. They started making out first, then we all started making out. Well, I asked them to make out. You know this was in high school so you could be very up front with girls if it was in a comfortable situation. I had one of the girls wrap her legs around the other girl's torso. The other one's making out with her, feeling the tits. I start banging her.

We're going at it, I'm doing the one girl and I hear the voice of my good friend, Larry. I look over and I see Larry and with some other guys like peaking in, watching us. And Larry is looking very intently to see if my shit is in there or if we're just dry humping. Larry's like, "Oh yeah. Yeah, yeah. It's in there guys." He starts clapping then they all start clapping. I'm doing the one girl then it was like, "OK, here we go," the other girl hops on. I've been tested since but this was all unprotected sex. We were pretty drunk. We finished up and then the second girl got out of the tub crying because apparently she liked me for real. So I think she was sitting there watching me with the first girl, getting very jealous and that's why she was willing to hop on.

I had hooked up with another girl in the hot tub the week before. But that was like four of us in the hot tub, girls and guys. As far as I knew, that time with me and the two girls was the first hot tub sex, unless the mother and father probably had done it.

The whole thing lasted maybe 15, 20 minutes until the one girl got fed up and couldn't handle being in her own head and went in the shower and freaked out. In retrospect I feel very bad about the whole situation because she was very upset. She wasn't very attractive. Her friend, the first one, was extremely attractive. When the second girl got out and ran into the shower I told the first girl, you know, let's go in there to try to talk it all out.

The one girl gave excellent blowjobs. That was the one who wasn't very attractive. That's how they always get you, you know what I mean? The real hot ones, they're the ones who just don't know how to do it. The sex itself was under water, it wasn't very pleasurable. It basically turned into, "Look guys! I'm having sex!" The shower was a little bit better because we kissed a little bit more but what was just because we were all wasted.

(...and how not to)

Later on that night I was sitting with the guy's dad who owned the place, feeling proud of myself and he played some AC/DC and this song called "Rasputin" by Boney M. It's a good song. I'll never forget that. The downside is that I was feeling proud of myself for doing a very horrible thing. I've grown up since then.

It was basically a disaster but at the same time I did lose my virginity to two girls in a hot tub. If they were in front of me right now and asked if I wanted to do it again, I would. But... I've forgiven myself and I've accepted absolution and I think I'm all right.

How to Lose Your Virginity

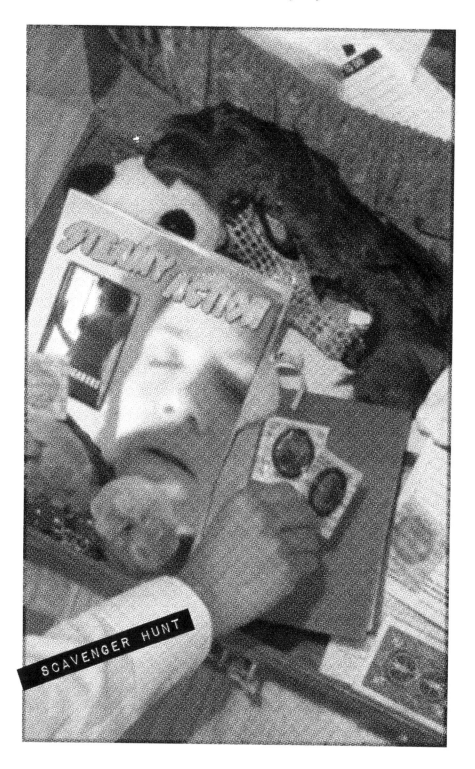

(...and how not to)

"HOW DO YOU PUT THESE THINGS ON?"

2

My memory on learning how to properly use a condom is hazy. I would like to say that I received my first lesson in high school health class. But I think the first time I witnessed a condom "used" was when a sex ed teacher demonstrated putting one on a banana in some movie, or it may have even been in an episode of *Beverly Hills 90210*. I can't remember exactly.

I can, however, say with some degree of confidence that my generation witnessed, grew up during, the condom explosion. Because of HIV/AIDS, the increase in teenage pregnancy, it made conversations about condoms imperative. I can recall when *SPIN* Magazine included a free condom in one of its issues, causing headlines and stirring up debate. I remember the first time I saw a commercial for Trojan condoms on MTV and people called it scandalous.

Nowadays free condoms are available on most college campuses and many high schools. The importance of protected sex has become so ingrained in our collective consciousness, even some bars leave them out. Condoms are part of the process, the experience, it's even part of the foreplay.

Here now are a few more reminders of the physically safe way to approach intercourse, in which condoms played an important role in the stories themselves.

THE ESCAPE CLAUSE
Derek, 30

I'm from Winston-Salem, North Carolina, maybe a four or five-hour drive from Myrtle Beach, South Carolina. It was a trip we'd make maybe on a quarterly basis. My friend Bob's parents owned a beach house there so a bunch of us 17-year-olds went to Myrtle Beach, which I guess would be an appropriate setting for some people to lose their virginity. Really it's just a very cheesy place.

There was me, Bob, Nate, Ed, and Terry. On the first night of a weekend trip we were hanging out on the beach smoking some dope and we met these girls who were about our age. Our buddy Terry was two years older than us and knew someone who could get us beer, or one of the girls was able to get us beers. Whoever got it, we took a bunch of beers to this girl's place where there wasn't any parental supervision.

I connected with this one girl and I was definitely nervous because I could see where the progression was going. I was still a virgin because I had just broken up with a girlfriend of two years who wanted to wait until marriage.

Everyone was playing a drinking game, which loosened me up a bit. I don't remember exactly what took us from that level to the next, but she said to me, "Let's go check out my room." We went to her room and started to hook up total high school style. I wanted to try to have sex but I didn't know if it was a possibility so I excused myself. I went up to Terry and asked him, "Do you have any condoms?" I go back to the room and we're finally making progress.

It gets to the point where we're naked and I think, "All right. It's all or nothing at this point." I put on the condom, make the move, and honest to God I lasted maybe nine seconds.

I don't know how I kept it together but I said, "Aw, shit. Hold on one second." She was just getting into it and she was like, "What? What?" Not knowing what to do, I stalled and blurted out, "I think the rubber broke."

I went back out to the living room and asked Terry, "Do you have another condom? He was like, "Why?" I was like, "Just give me another condom if you have one," thinking I could buy enough time to work myself back up. I got another condom and went back to the room but I had lost it. It so wasn't going to happen. The girl just looked at me and asked, "Do you want to go out and play the rest of the drinking game?" It was the greatest thing she could have said to me. I didn't know how to segue out of there but she did it for me and let me off the hook.

> Some Japanese condoms are a little bit smaller and a lot of guys in Japan will sort of brag secondhand about the size of their penis by saying they have to order their condoms over the Internet. But you can find international condoms in any convenience store.
>
> *Stan, 26*
> *Kumamoto, Japan*

(...and how not to)

PHANTOM SHOPPER
Patrick, 25

This was in Hillsboro, New Jersey. We were in marching band together. She was in the color guard and I played trumpet. She was a year older than me and I was a freshman. It was that classic "I loved her at first sight" kind of thing – my first real infatuation.

We eventually started dating and by the end of my sophomore year I was anxious to lose mine. She was kind of hesitant about it since she lost hers a couple years before.

But I kept working on her and around the time I thought something was close to happening, and this is the best part of the story: I was with my younger brother who was in eighth grade and we were driving down the main route in town. I pulled into the local pharmacy and I was like, "Little brother, you got to do me a favor. I need you to go in there and buy me condoms." I wasn't about to do it myself – I had a little brother here to do it for me.

He actually had no problem with it. You know, little brother – big brother kind of thing, a good little brother deed. So he goes in, and I waited in the car the whole time. He comes out and says, "Pat, you're not going to believe what just happened." I was like, "What did you get 'em?" He said, "Oh, I got 'em. And I turned around and my religion teacher was in line right behind me." She didn't say anything, just gave him the look. He wasn't mad about it, I think in a way he appreciated the experience – buying condoms for his older brother and getting caught by his religious studies teacher.

Then later that week I went over to her house, condoms in hand, and she said, "Yeah, tonight's the night," so of course I was a nervous wreck. I didn't tell her the story about my brother, she probably would have made me wait a few more months as punishment. Like I said I was nervous because she already lost her virginity. I was fumbling for awhile and it was your basic *American Pie* kind of thing. We were just making out for awhile and then she was absolutely silent for the rest of our sexual experience. She really wasn't into it. A very "laid there" type of girl.

She comforted me a bit because I honestly lasted like 60 seconds. I was like, "I'm sorry. Was it OK?" She was like, "It's OK, Pat. It was all right."

I think my brother eventually asked me if the condoms were the right kind. I said, "I guess. I don't know."

So having my little brother buy the condoms was the best part of the whole story. It opened him up pretty early to the idea of buying condoms.

BY THE BOOK
Nora, 30

I was a senior in high school and I was about to graduate when I met this older guy through a friend who was dating a friend of his. He was 23 years old. We hooked up and just drank, nothing intellectual, just a party scene. I had been a real advocate of using condoms and I was the one who always told my friends, "Don't get sick." At 15, 16 years old I was abstaining but all the while passing out condoms to my sexually active friends.

My mother was a child psychologist so from an early age she told me pretty much everything that could go wrong with sex. Not so much go wrong with it but all of the ramifications of being unsafe about it. The one thing she didn't warn me about was older guys. But I kind of had my mind made up that I wanted to get it over with. All my friends had lost their virginity and I just wanted to get it done. It wasn't something that was supposed to be romantic. It was like driving for the first time when you get your license. At some point you have sex.

So I guess I had known this guy for a week and we did it. I told him it was my first time and I insisted that he wore a condom, which he was not happy about. It wasn't fun at all, it was painful. He was unrelenting about how un-sexual I was. But it being my first time, I didn't know how to be sexual. I didn't have an orgasm but at least it was "mission accomplished".

He was enormous. He was huge and it hurt like hell and it wasn't fun. And everything you hear about big dicks being great, nope. They're not. They're hell.

I don't regret it not being like an intimate moment. I was glad that I did use a condom because a lot of my friends were pregnant, like three out of five of my friends were pregnant by 17. I had tried giving safe sex advice to all my friends but some of them just didn't understand the importance or had the concept of being careful.

Like six in the morning and I was sleeping and my parents unlocked my door and snuck in. At first I thought it was a dream, but I woke up to my parents rapping about anti-sex or like safe sex and the importance of using condoms. My mom and dad were wearing backwards hats, my dad had his arms crossed like Run DMC and was beatboxing. My mom had this crib sheet she was rapping off of. It was something ridiculous like, "We love you son. Don't be dumb. If you have sex, use a condom."

Kevin, 22
Atlantic City, New Jersey

(...and how not to)

THE PRESENT
Bud, 27

I still have this leather wallet that I've had for about 10 years now. I got it when I was 17. This would have been the semester before I graduated from high school – so I guess like the fall semester of my senior year.

    I had a girlfriend and we hadn't had sex but we'd been dating for awhile. I wanted to have sex really bad and she was hesitant. Then as sort of an early graduation present she gave me a wallet and it was weird to get a wallet as a graduation present. I was thinking well that's nice. Then she told me, "But there's more to it. Look inside." I opened the wallet and she had put a condom inside it, which was her way of saying that we could have sex.

    It was funny, it wasn't very sexy but more just comic and funny because we were both, "Oh, I don't really know what to do." Neither of us were more of the "expert" than the other, which was good. I just remember it as being funny and like it's the only time you were allowed to laugh that much while having sex and it be OK. After that you're supposed to get more sophisticated. You know, you're not really allowed to laugh that much, especially when you're having sex with someone new for the first time. For some unspoken reason it has to be deadly serious or it has to somehow be really passionate. But for the very first time it was OK to laugh because there was no expectation that anybody would really know what they were doing. That made it better, I think. It made it more relaxed.

    I can remember, with that girl, later on having sex seven times in one night. Nothing like that has ever happened to me after that. And I think the reason is that you were able to be funny and have fun when you're new to it. There was nothing really riding on it so it was more like both people were able to see it as something cute or fun.

SCAVENGER HUNT
Aaron, 27

I went to an all-boys boarding school in Virginia and I met a girl my senior year who went to an all-girls boarding school about two hours south of me. We continued to date after I started college, still having not slept together. So I was in college, and I would go and visit her some weekends and it happened that her roommate's family lived in the town where this boarding school was. When I would go to visit her, her roommate's family let me stay with them.

    We had been talking about, you know, sleeping together, and etcetera and there was one particular night where her roommate's family signed her off of campus and we went back to her roommate's house and the family was away. We were left alone in the house.

We sort of agreed, "OK, well... we'll make love tonight if we can find a condom in the house." So the two of us scoured the entire place and it took about two hours. We went through everything, the mom's underwear drawer, the whole nine yards and we're not finding one. After about two hours of searching we were in her roommate's younger brother's room and we find a suitcase under his bed filled with about five or six porn videos, a bunch of dirty magazines, and a full box of condoms. That was when I lost my virginity, my freshman year of college when we basically stole a condom.

We were there for the night by ourselves so it was actually really beautiful. It was great.

> We were so nervous about throwing away the condom in her dad's garbage that we went out about a half a mile from her house into the woods, dug a hole and buried the condom. We buried it like a foot deep, like we were burying a body in *The Sopranos* or something.
>
> Art, 27
Washington, D.C.

60, 59, 58, 57, 56...
Melanie, 24

I was a late bloomer, 21 years old. Doug and I were members of the same co-ed, community service fraternity. After our friendship transitioned rather smoothly into a relationship, we found out that both of us were still virgins.

Eight months into us dating we had that ridiculous talk... "Um, I guess we're going to have sex sometime." But I was all, "I'm not ready!" And he's like, "Neither am I!" He was a year older than me and when he graduated he moved to an apartment and I'd leave school to visit him on weekends.

The first time it almost happened he had guests and we thought, "Oh, we can't do it because Linda and Don are on the other side of the door. Oh no." He also said he didn't have any condoms and I told him, "Yeah, you're not having any sex without any condoms." When I got back to school I went to the health center where they handed out the free ones and I pretended to be an R.A. saying I needed condoms for my entire floor. I scored a box of 60.

That next weekend we finally did it and we counted backwards from 60. So the first condom was 60 and then the next time it was like, "Better get number 59." That morning after, he took me out for a breakfast at McDonald's because I really liked McDonald's breakfasts. He probably thought I was such a cheap date.

I still have some of those first box of condoms. We broke up before he and I could count all the way down to condom number one. But that's when it happened. At the time we were in a loving and committed relationship and it was a really good experience.

(…and how not to)

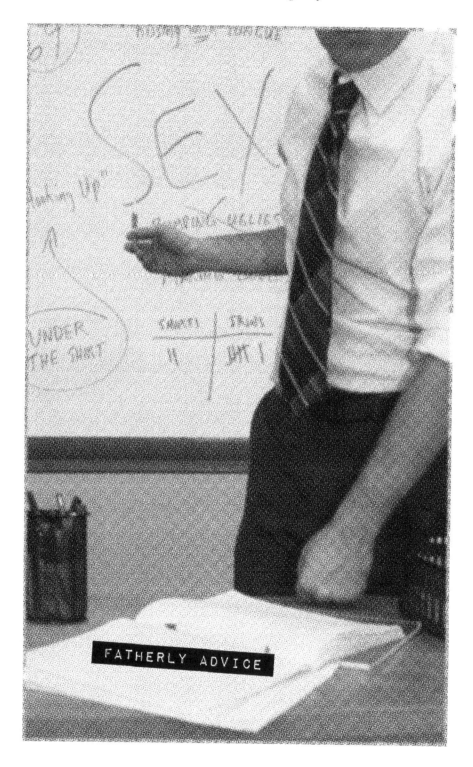

(...and how not to)

"PENIS IS THE PROPER WORD... VULVA IS THE PROPER WORD."

3

The above quote is taken from a sexual educational video – a free rental that my mother forced me to watch when I was 12. I unwillingly sat through the VHS puberty lesson and a folk singer appeared on the screen, sitting in a playground and strumming a miniature guitar while singing a song about the proper names for the male and female anatomy. I, in turn, took that song back to school where it became an in-joke amongst my friends: penis is the proper word - vulva is the proper word.

In sexual education there was the tendency to laugh at the situation, vocabulary words, etc. But when presented with the real thing in the bedroom, fear and apprehension is a far more common response than laughter. As much as you can try to prepare with book smarts, there is no substitute for hands-on experience.

This next collection of stories represents a heightened sense of awareness about the workings of the opposite sex, or sex in general, as a result of the first time. Lessons learned about who they were, what they liked, what they didn't like, what to do, and what not to do.

STUDYING A "BROAD"
George, 24

I was going to school in London. I was dating a girl, my first girlfriend, who wouldn't sleep with me. She was back in the States. We broke up over the phone and that same night I met a girl from Denmark.

Europeans do things differently; they're more open about sex. Her being from Denmark and me being from the U.S., we knew that we weren't going to be in the same place for very long. We had sex three times and then she left the country. That was it. I still keep in contact with her, email every so often.

It was interesting because I kind of assumed that the way I would lose it is that a girl would finally say, "Let's have sex." I learned that's not the way things happen. I initiated and she said, "Sure." That's how I've been doing it ever since. Guys have to initiate.

THE GAME
Anthony, 23

All right. The time when I lost my virginity was Dec. 24th, 1998. I was a spring chicken. A fresh boy straight out of the coop. And it was a black piece of pussy that just had my name on it. She was smokin'.

I was the ever-present wingman for one of my friends going out with her. So I was the personality, he was the physicality. And finally I just talked the bitch into it. She dropped him and then went for me. You got to trick a girl. The way to get pussy is to trick a bitch. Trick a bitch!

Basically I've been tricking girls ever since I got my first piece of ass and I will remain tricking girls until I find a woman who is right for me. I will tell them what I have to tell them to get them in the sack.

You can be a fat, nothing, white kid who really has no business getting any butt, or you can get a lot of ass if you act like the number one stud. And you always do this, that's how you should always think and act. So when a girl comes up to you and wants to have sex with you don't look surprised, even though she could be hot and you're a slob. You just go with it and that's how you trick it.

So a little, chubby white boy like myself didn't know what I was in for. She came by and we made passionate love under the Christmas tree until my mother came home. My mother walked in the house and found us both half naked so it of course broke up the proceedings. But that is the story of how I, a little white boy with jungle fever, lost my virginity.

Look, the fact of the matter is, if you really want to get what you want, you gotta trick them. Trick them into thinking you're sweet and nice. Because if you tell them the truth, she ain't gonna want your ass. You're really not that ill, just remember that. If you're not tricking her, then you're gettin' tricked.

(...and how not to)

> Losing your virginity is the worst for girls. For guys it's like heaven.
>
> *Lisa, 30*
> *Austin, Texas*

RANDOM BOYS
Vanessa, 25

A couple days after my 13th birthday, I was at the mall with my best friend. This guy came up to me and said, "You're cute. What's your number?" Being that I was young and insecure, something as simple as a guy asking for my number made me feel cool, I gave it to him. He was older, maybe 20. I told him I was 17. Whether or not he believed me, he was like, "Come over to my house."

My friend and I got into his car and she and I pretty much knew what was going to happen once we got there. I started to prepare myself for the inevitable because I knew once I got to his house it would be too late to back down.

I never said I didn't want to do it, so it happened up in his bed. My friend and one of his friends did it in another room. That's how we knew it was kind of a set-up, because some other guy was already there waiting for us. Getting us girls there was a plan and it felt like a plan. That sucks when it's your first experience.

I was a 13-year-old insecure little girl who felt fat and ugly. He was the first guy who ever asked for my phone number so when he first came up to me I felt pretty special. After it happened, I didn't feel special at all. These guys wouldn't even go out of their way to drop us off. We had to take the bus. The whole bus ride home my friend and I talked about it, about how neither of us liked it, neither of us thought it felt good. It wasn't the right way. It wasn't right at all. It wasn't right until four years later when I dated my first serious boyfriend.

I learned a lot from that experience though. It was my first introduction into the male mind and I learned to forever avoid going over random boys' houses.

> I gave her a call three weeks later. I wasn't in San Francisco anymore, but I was willing to go back to meet her. I don't think she appreciated that very much so I've learned that one of the hardest things for a guy is knowing when to call back afterwards if you want to hook up again. I can say that three weeks is definitely too long.
>
> *Gary, 26*
> *Brissie, Australia*

THE HETEROSEXUAL LITMUS TEST
Betsy, 19

I like guys and girls but I was trying to decide which I liked more. I was kind of more into girls but I came from a real Mormon family. They kind of know I'm gay now but it's unspoken. It's not admitted. So I was going to give it one last shot to see if I could settle down with a guy before I dated girls full-time and cause a family upheaval. Basically I had sex with a guy to find out how straight or not I was, and it helped me figure out that I wasn't.

I met this guy at a random party. I was kind of into him, kind of not, and we started dating casually. One night we go to this concert and he has some ecstasy so we eat a bunch of X. We spend all night rolling together. Next morning we woke up and I thought, "OK. What the fuck? Let's see how this works." I tried and I didn't get off. We dated for another four weeks and I just never got into it.

Matt always wanted to have sex in the morning. It was hard to go through because I could see him and all his manliness and it bothered me. I couldn't turn off the lights and pretend he was a girl. He ended up dumping me and I was upset for about two days and then felt relieved because I was free to date women.

I did like Matt; I cared about him as a person. He was awesome and we had a lot in common. He was a pianist and I play the piano too. I fell in love with the boy on an emotional and intellectual level. Physically… the sex was not as enjoyable as it should be.

The whole complex of losing your virginity after growing up in a Mormon household is built up a lot. Mormons actually call premarital sex the worst sin second to murder. So in the hierarchy of sin, you can murder someone and then the next worst thing you can do after that is have sex outside of marriage. So yeah, it's a huge deal. After I lost it, it didn't seem like a big deal at all. It helped me figure out what sex is really about. Like sex can't be about the relationship or about getting them to like you. Sex has to be about how you feel about them. And it appears I can only feel that way about other girls.

I'm glad it wasn't an *American Pie*-esque exchange of, "I love you" for having sex. I somehow managed to say, "I love you" a few weeks after having sex. I wouldn't have minded saying, "I love you" earlier; it was just very important to me that those two events not happen at the same time, because I felt like it would have been some sort of bizarre prostitution of exchanging one thing for the other.

Drew, 21
Metuchen, New Jersey

(...and how not to)

THE MOVE
Roy, 44

I was away on holiday with my brother and his friends in Mallorca on a two-week package tour. On the second night there I left a disco with this English girl. I literally just ended up with her. She pulled me into a field, pulled my trousers down and gave me a blowjob. Then she pulled me on top and I rid' her.

The one thing I remember is she tickled my balls, which was unbelievable... the balls. That was just something else, you never would have expected that.

She was English, I'm Irish. She was 17 and I was 15. I went back home to my girlfriend after that and I was a different man. I was ready for sex.

We never traded numbers or nothing, it was just all about the riding. It was excellent. I'm actually embarrassed that I don't know her name. But she was short with blonde hair. She wasn't great looking but she was all right looking. She was nice and funny and nice to talk to. And she tickled my balls... that was the big thing, tickling the balls, man. That made my ears wiggle.

FATHERLY ADVICE
Leif, 22

The first time was with a hippie chick. She was quite a hippie so naturally she was... natural down there. Quite a forest scene down there. I wasn't ready to go down on her, couldn't handle the oral thing so I figure we'll get into some regular penetration. I put the rubber on, started going at it and five, maybe ten minutes into it, the condom kind of got wrapped up in some of her hairs there and sort of got whipped right off. I had heard that it's possible for condoms to slip off inside and that's what I figured had happened, but when I looked down and saw the actual entanglement situation, I was a little disturbed. It broke the mood for awhile. We hung out for a bit, smoked some weed, then got back into it after about a half hour or so.

It finished well for me but I did have to do some mouth work on her after the fact to make sure she was satisfied. My father once gave me some advice that I've always tried to follow. He and I were in the garage sharing a cigarette and drinking some whiskey and he just randomly said, "You should never enter a woman unless she's had at least two orgasms." He's a smart man, works in home health care so he's got a mind for knowing what people need and getting it taken care of.

It's easy for a man to get off whereas women, there's more work involved. If you're going to get off, you might as well put in the work beforehand. So I made sure by the end of the night she at least had two.

THE INSTRUCTION MANUAL
Mark, 21

I was eighteen and my girlfriend at the time and I were at my dad's house in Cape Cod, Massachusetts. She had done it before, which felt weird. I was really kind of nervous, like a stage fright sort of feeling. It wasn't like a losing-an-erection type of nervous but it was a definite intense anxiety. But she was extremely patient with me. Before, during, and after the act there was feedback and instructions. She was a feminist organization leader at Penn State and coincidentally a very good sex coach.

One of the things she told me was that a lot of guys will tend to just thrust downward: up and down, up and down. That doesn't really stimulate the clitoris. The way she described it was, for guys it feels good when they're pushing down, but for girls it feels good when the guy is pushing up. She got me moving in that motion and she was right. It's made all the difference in my experiences with her and every girl I've been with after her. I'm not bragging but girls tend to like that better than the "Wham, bam, thank you ma'am" type of thrusts.

Losing my virginity was a little bit of a bigger thing than I thought it would be. It's an important physical kind of rite of passage of sorts. And you want to do it well, you want to do it right.

We did it that first time and it was fun, but it's a difficult thing to separate the anxiety of the whole situation out of it. The next time we did it, and I know this sounds counter-intuitive since guys are horny all the time, but honestly I was still nervous about having sex. But with her help I acclimated to it and she was a good coach.

LIKE A WALK IN THE PARK
Ann Marie, 31

I was 13 and I lost my virginity at a carnival, like a little street fair in my neighborhood, to a boy that was actually a… OK, he was a carnie. And I lost my virginity in a broken, unused tilt-a-whirl car inside the back of a semi truck. For some reason I just thought that was the biggest, greatest idea because you know, you're in middle school and everybody's talking about boy-girl stuff. And I was just, "Well what's the big deal? I'll just go do it." And so I found the quickest, easiest route and it was a little carnie kid who was 16, just hittin' his puberty and I think he may have lost his virginity that day too because it sucked. Not that it ever got better for me 'cause I'm not about the guys. I can't remember exactly the name of the festival or where it was located. To be honest, being 31 now, I try to block it out sometimes.

(...and how not to)

The kid was working on the tilt-a-whirl ride. The whole thing was his idea. He was like, "Well, you know my boss isn't here. I got a place for us to go." I don't have a clue who he had running the tilt-a-whirl cars when he wasn't there. Those people must have been on that tilt-a-whirl ride for like a good 10 minutes, not even 'cause it was like maybe a five-minute walk to the semi truck and then it took 30 seconds long and then we walked back. The walk was pretty much the whole duration of the time we were gone. I mean it was like barely touching one another. He wasn't even a one-minute man. That's how I lost mine and I promised myself that I wouldn't do it again 'cause it was just horrible. I tried with a few other boys and then I met the first woman that I slept with and then it dawned on me, "Yeah, I'm not supposed to be having sex with boys ever. I'm supposed to be a boy."

So a couple years later I met the first woman I slept with. I was in a park and she was rollerblading and she ended up falling near me and I helped her get up.

She kept saying that her ankle was hurt and I was like, "OK, it'll be all right. I'll help you to your car. Maybe you should go to the hospital." I could care less, to be honest. I just wanted to leave with this pretty girl. I was like, "Sweet. She's got a convertible and she's pretty. I'll sit in the car with her." Well we didn't end up at the hospital. We ended up at her place. There wasn't anything about her that said lesbian, specifically. There's just that thing inside you that says, "This is one I could hit on."

In the car I was kind of like playing around with her neck and telling her, "Oh, it's going to be OK. We'll get to the hospital." Then I was like, "Oh, I bet you have your own place." She was about 12 years older than me. I was like, "I bet it's cool having your own place." She's like, "Well, yeah." And I was like, "Maybe I should see it sometime." "Well, we could go there now." I was like, "Sweet. I'm ready."

In all honesty I barely ever count the first time on the tilt-a-whirl as the actual time because it did absolutely nothing for my sexual development whatsoever. It was just something that closeted me more. But as far as with the woman that I slept with, I just remember feeling a big sigh of relief.

It was clumsy, but it was good. I was like, "I think I know how to take off pantyhose." I ripped them off. I was good at that." I mean, I can't get the crap on but I can get the shit off.

And it dawned on me that guys weren't really what I was wanting. It was one of those things where, your first time you hope that you feel like you're on cloud nine, and it should be totally exhilarating and that's what my first time with a woman was like.

She gave me a ride home, at which point my dad asked me, "Who was that?" I was like, "I don't know." "Then how did you get in her car?" "I... I don't know, Dad. I don't. I have no clue." And I hid in my bedroom for the next few days. I was a little creeped out afterward. When I was growing up you generally didn't really talk about stuff like that when I was growing up. So I didn't really exactly know how to define what happened so I went into hiding, kept a little to myself until eventually I decided, "That was good. I want to do it again." I was a little monster from that moment on and hitting on girls at the mall and taking girls home. Then I went to college and that was a free-for-all.

REFLECTIONS
Tiffany, 29

I explain first time sex as a pain you can take. And you do it over and over and over again until you're good at it. My boyfriend was 19 and he had a very big cock.

It happened in his bedroom on his waterbed. At 16 I was truly too immature to have sex. When I went home I looked in the mirror and I thought, "Do I look different? Are people going to notice? Are people gonna think I look cool? Am I a woman? Is this normal?"

I called him up crying because of course I started to bleed. We talked and he was sweet about it.

ALL-NATURAL LUBRICANT
Kristen, 30

I was not necessarily conned into it but... I was. I was 18 and I wanted to make sure I turned 18 before I did it. I had had earlier opportunities but I wanted to wait until I was a little older. I was saving it for a graduation gift to myself.

I had been dating Rob for awhile, through most of high school. I was like, "Well I want to move to the next step." We go to the beach: Wildwood, New Jersey. We were sharing this beach house with two other couples and a single guy. There was a room with two double beds and there was another room with a single bed and pull-out couch.

Rob wanted to do it while we were at the beach house, and I thought, "After all these weeks, he finally wants to get down and busy and I'm on my period." He told me, "You really should do it now because it will hurt less." He was saying if you've never done it before, it will hurt the least if you do it when you have your period because, "Your period, it's like lubrication." He gave me this whole story. I was like, "Yeah but it's gonna be messy."

He sounded real convincing and he said the hotel staff would clean it up. I was duped from the beginning. I thought it was the right thing to do, the right time to do it. Maybe not right then when I was on my period, but Rob convinced me otherwise.

We were sharing this room with other people so we were trying to do it quick and not get caught. We were doing it and the bed broke and fell to the floor. The sheets were a wreck.

Everyone else eventually walked in and the bed is half on the floor, the sheets are off and wadded up in a ball in the corner. My girlfriend was like, "Ohmigod, you finally had sex?" And I'm like, "Yeah." And I told her about the whole period thing and she's like, "What are you dumb?" And I was like, "Yeah." She's like, "You never have sex on your period." I was like, "Rob said it wouldn't hurt as bad and it would be more slippery. He said it would feel better." That's what the dude said. He also said that the senses would be heightened.

Boys will tell you anything to get you in bed. At least it was safe sex.

(...and how not to)

A SAD STORY ABOUT SOMETHING THAT MEANT NOTHING
Mary, 22

I was in a juvenile program for kids on drugs and stuff. I wasn't on drugs. For whatever reason my mom was fine with her other kids, she just didn't want me. She worked for the state of Oregon and, through connections, managed to get me in.

I came home for Mother's Day weekend and my mom went off on me on how she didn't want me there and how she wished I would have really made her Mother's Day special by not coming home at all. She said she wished she'd never had me, just went off. I didn't have anywhere to go. It was a small town, I was depressed and I had to get away. My older sister's friend Tim lived nearby. I just needed somewhere to go, someone to talk to. I was 15 and he was 19.

I walked over to his house and he acted comforting, he talked to me and calmed me down. We were sitting on his bed and I was crying and everything. He just totally pulled my strings and took advantage of the situation. It happened very quickly. I'm pretty sure I heard him say he was a virgin too but I can't be sure if he really was or if that was just part of his story to get his pants off.

Afterwards he walked me outside and told me, "You know we're not together, right? This meant nothing." I said, "Yeah, I know," and I walked home by myself. It wasn't exactly rape. I didn't want to do it but, then again, I never said yes. And I wasn't expecting us to be together or fall in love just because we had sex. I wasn't one of those girls but for him to say that so bluntly just sucked.

My sister was my best friend and she saw I was balling. I had gone over to Tim's to escape but all it did was make the depression even worse so I told her what happened. She said she wouldn't tell anybody but she was pissed because she liked him. After I went back to the juvenile home she told everybody.

My mom found out about a year later. I was back home, again on Mother's Day and again she was bitching me out for something and offhandedly stated, "At least all my kids are still virgins." I shouted, "Fuck you. I'm not a virgin." I told her what happened and how it happened on the last Mother's Day and how it was her fault, "There's your fucking Mother's Day gift, you stupid bitch." She called me a whore. I shouldn't have gone there but she set me off with those things she said about her darling kids being virgins. We don't go at it like that anymore but we're still not close.

I wished I would have done it some other way. I wanted to stay a virgin until I was married and get married in a Mormon temple. It killed me that I would miss out on that. I started drinking and since I already did it once, I lost my self-respect and became a hoochie mama there for awhile. It ruined me for a good year or two but I've matured since then and realized that some people just suck.

The way I lost my virginity affected my sex life for years and years after that. I strongly believe that, especially for women, sex is definitely more mental and emotional. If you have a bad experience, you really can't enjoy sex. It took a whole five years after my first time until I was able to have any pleasure from sex whatsoever.

I was dating this guy, we were sexually active for 10 months and I only got off once that whole 10 months. They say good sex makes up only 20% of a relationship but bad sex takes up 70% of it and that's one of the main reasons I broke up with the guy. It's like my first time ruined me and I was emotionally scarred from it. I just stopped having sex altogether until finally I fell in love and then *boom* – sex was awesome.

If I ever have a daughter, she's going to be the first to know that it needs to be something special or he should at least be important to you or it can scar you. You live and learn and every experience gives you more strength. And you never know, if I hadn't gone through that experience I might not be where I am now, so I wouldn't necessarily change it if I could... but I might.

UNCLE KNOWS BEST
Corey, 34

I was cruising down the back roads of Michigan on my Honda Spree. I'm minding my own business then I see this girl in a Bon Jovi, stone-washed jean jacket with the fringe, walking along the side of the road. I was 15, this probably would have been in 1988.

I whip up next to her like I'm on a Harley or something instead of my little scooter, and I say, "Hey. What's going on?" She's like, "Going to the store to get some smokes." So I'm like, "Sweet. Want a ride?" like hop on my fucking tiny Honda Spree. It was the first time I rode with someone else on that scooter and it could barely take off. It was bogged down so I had to run along side it to get it moving.

Finally I get the thing going fast enough so we won't tip over. We're going down maybe a mile and she starts feeling my stomach. Then she reaches around and grabs my package, I'm like, "Whoa." "Pull over," she says. In Michigan there's a lot of like two-tracks where you can just peel off into the woods. We find someplace secluded and start kissing.

We lay down in the dirty, sticky pine needles. I get on top of her and she takes just one of her legs out of her Palmettos, not even Guess jeans, but like the cheap Palmettos. At this point in my life I had not even jacked off. This was it, this was the very first. We're doing it and it was the weirdest thing, my leg cramped up and my body seized and all this stuff came out of my penis and got all over the place. It felt really good but I was alarmed by it.

We got dressed and I drove her to the gas station and I didn't even get her name. She got cigarettes and I filled my tank and I peeled off. I was still freaking out about the orgasm. AIDS was still mysterious and scary to me and I didn't know if stuff coming out meant something was wrong. I didn't know. So I went home and I couldn't tell my dad so I called the only person I knew I could talk to about this: my mom's brother, Uncle Lenny.

Uncle Lenny is totally super cool. I'm 34 and he's 75 now and he still gets all the chicks. Really laid back and he's kind of connected to the Detroit underground. I knew he was the guy who could give me some insight into what went down. I told him the situation and said, "I don't know what happened. This like pus stuff came out of my penis." He was like, "You never jacked off before?" I said, "No." He was like, "Get into the tub. Draw a hot bath. Burp the worm for a few minutes and tell me if that stuff comes out again."

I followed his instructions, got in the tub, jacked off; it felt good and I was like, "Oh, awesome." For some reason it all made sense to me.

(...and how not to)

REACHING FOR NIRVANA
Emil, 36

Back in high school, in North Austin, sex wasn't the first thing on my mind but I always wondered when it would happen. At the time I was more concerned with making a lot of money and a friend of mine and I created a business... well... manufacturing ecstasy. He actually got in trouble for it. I, by chance, missed out on any repercussions.

This was back right when ecstasy first started to get big. That was my thing in high school. I would go to a party, hang out. I always had girlfriends but I never slept with anybody, and the first girl I ever wanted to really sleep with, we talked about it, she was uncomfortable with it and I was like, "OK. Not a problem."

As I started straightening out, stopped selling and trying to turn a new leaf, I became a Buddhist and my best friend at that time, Owen, his mother was Buddhist. That's how I was exposed to it, through her. We had talked about how the biggest things you could do that are wrong were stealing and lying. I never stole anything, I never lied about anything. I sold drugs, I did a lot of things that were really fucked up according to societal views but according to her she's like, "There's nothing wrong with that."

We would chant together, we'd smoke pot, get high, hang out. She told me, "Anything that you chant for, you'll be able to get." And this woman was the most incredibly beautiful woman I had ever met before. She was married, she was my best friend's mother, not to mention my family's next door neighbor. My parents didn't really talk to their family because my parents were hard-core fucking Episcopalians - different worlds. But I would go over to that house all the time and I'd chant and... and all I ever wanted... I wanted to be with her. Was her husband going to have a problem with it? I didn't know. That wasn't an issue as far as stealing or lying. He was a vice president for a pretty major international financial conglomerate, so he was never home.

Months had gone by since I started chanting and there were other girls that I had been with, made out with. I went down on girls, girls went down on me and you know, according to whatever you think sex is. Had I had sex? Not really. Every single time the possibility of sex came up, you know, they were hesitant. It's like OK, not a problem. I wasn't out to hurt somebody. If they didn't feel comfortable with sex then that's cool. We'll drink and hang out, we'll have fun, we'll take some X. We don't have to have sex, we can do other things. Kissing and touching was great but at the same time, these were young girls. Loretta on the other hand was a woman and incredibly beautiful. And every day she's all I'd ever fucking chant for.

Then one day, I'm at the house and her son Owen and our other friend Jay were like, "We're gonna go out and do some military maneuvers and sleep out in the woods." They were hardcore into playing D&D but they also liked to go out and do weird covert operations and fuckin' sneak around people's backyards. I was like, "All right dude. I'm just going to spend the night at your house. You know, if that's cool with you."

They left and Loretta said I could watch a movie with her in her bedroom. So we're sitting there watching a movie, the movie that actually later on got me thinking of joining the Navy... *An Officer and a Gentleman*. And there's some steamy parts in it.

How to Lose Your Virginity

She's in her bed and I'm lying on the floor and she says, "You can lie on my bed if you want to." So now I'm lying in her bed and she had always told me how attractive she thought I was. She never looked at me as though I was the type of person her son was, running around in the woods playing war games. She thought I was very mature. Nobody else was there. Her son was gone, her husband was gone. It started with her putting her hand on my arm and we made love for hours. I had thought, from the time I was 12 years old until the time I was 15 years old, about sex with girls but I knew it wouldn't be a pleasurable experience for them so I never wanted to go through with it. Not to say that it was a religious experience but the fact remains that it did enlighten me spiritually... it was incredible. And she was my spiritual teacher, as well as my sexual one.

Nobody knew what I was chanting for. Her son didn't know what I was chanting for. I wasn't gonna tell Owen that I wanted to do it with his mom. Chanting and praying for what you want, it's inside of yourself. As far as the prayer goes, you're not verbally asking out loud, it's just the heart's desire that is inside of you, what you want. To actually be with her after wanting that for so long it was very spiritual. And every time that I've been with anyone else after that you know, I always looked at sex as a spiritual event as opposed to just having sex... just doing whatever with anybody.

All my buddies growing up, they'd screw whoever. They didn't care about people's feelings or emotions. But for me, if I'm to learn how to make love to a woman, I need to learn from a woman.

Owen found out about it though. Our buddy Jay told him. Because... once again... high school, these guys were trying to have sex with whoever and whatever and Jay was sleeping with this girl Donna and he'd never been with anybody before so he was always pre-ejaculating all over her. But Donna also had a crush on me and so she and I later on slept together but because I'd already slept with Loretta it was like I knew what I needed to do to make this something enjoyable for her as opposed to just concentrating on how I was going to get off. Donna had told me what happened with Jay and wondered why I didn't have the same problem. I was like, "Well I need to tell you something. I slept with Owen's mom." And so high school still being high school, she told Jay and Jay told Owen and Owen confronted me during our high school graduation.

He was all right with it. His mother was married to his stepfather so she had obviously had several different men in her life before. He wasn't upset with me but he was weird about it. But what can you do? It wasn't like she was drunk, I didn't take advantage of her. If anything she took advantage of me. She stayed married to her husband and I don't think he ever found out. But it was great. And it wasn't like something she did all the time, sleeping with a bunch of young guys. I waited for the longest time and then when it happened for me it was... it was religious.

(see page 221)

(...and how not to)

BIG BROTHER KNOWS ALL THE TRICKS
DJ Ronrific, 33

I'm originally from St. Joseph, Missouri. Been out in Denver for about the past 20 years. I left the "Show-Me State" when I was like eight years old, moved up here to Colorado and lived in a suburb of Denver called Arvada. It's predominantly, I'd say, 95% white.

The first time I kissed a girl I was about 13 years old. Kissing pretty much just lead to other things, you know touchy-touchy, feel-feel... experimenting. She was my neighbor and her name was Charity. We always played downstairs at my house. Pretty much how it started out was like with most kids, "Let's play doctor."

It stopped there for a couple weeks and we went back to just being friends. Then one day it came down to it. We're back in my basement, that's where Mom always sent us kids, you know, "Go down there and play." So we're down there playing around and it was me, Charity, and two of our other neighborhood friends. We had a pool table and we were playing pool or whatever. Anyway me and her got to wrestling and it led me to getting an erection. She could feel it which got her kind of curious, but also kind of scared. We were both scared, shocked. We're still wrestling around and things and we started kissing. Then I started feeling on her and she was happy with that and now we're both really horny.

The other couple was still in the basement and they were laughing and kissing and doing their thing. They were pretty much boyfriend and girlfriend so they were in their own corner.

Charity and I got to rubbing on each other more and then pants came off so I started rubbing it on her vagina. That got her hot and I was hot too. I'm trying to get in there she's helping me at the same time. I'm so erect and she pretty much gets the head in for me. We're both virgins, you know, so of course she's tight. So anyway I get the head in a little bit and to make a long story short... after I got the head in after a good minute, I was done. That's it, all of it down. My virginity was broke, hers was partially broke because she experienced something, but she didn't get to climax like I did.

So we're sitting there underneath the pool table and she's like, "Oh, wow." And we got semen everywhere and we were freaked out about that. And we're looking at each other all crazy 'cause for one thing it's a black guy with a white female, plus she was new to the neighborhood. She had never had a black friend or even talked to a black guy before.

We were kind of distant toward each other and a couple of weeks down the road, eventually we were in the basement shooting pool again and the pants came down.

I had had a talk with my older brother and he told me to slow it down a bit to make it feel better for her. He was 18 so of course he knew. He was like, "Aw man, it happens to every male." So he gave me a little knowledge, you know slow it down, kiss on and rub on her clitoris and rub on her boobs and things. And I'm like, "Clitoris!? Wow! I'm 13." You know they gave us a little bit of sex education, but they just said how to make babies, they didn't say how to make it feel good.

So I get to rubbing on things and I'm taking his advice and I'm concentrating so much on what he told me to do, so my erection went away. I get to rubbing on her vagina and everything and I didn't know it but I found the clitoris and I felt her jump and she's like, "Huhhhh!" You know like, "Ooh, what was that?" It kind of shocked her a little bit. Body kind of clenched and shivered. *Bam!* New discovery... for me and her. Of course she knew what it was, it's on her body. But this was the first time she felt someone else touch it.

So now I'm rubbing on that and everything and kissing on her titties and things. It pretty much got me erect again, so I'm like, "Wow, I got to try to not bust a nut so quick like I did last time." So I get down there and I'm rubbing and I'm so erect I can't really get in cause she's so tight. I had to have her take her two fingers and try to hold her snapper open, her vagina. So she kind of opened it a little bit and I'm rubbing on there and I get the head in, and it got in a little easier this time. And she's draining on me, you know, and I'm like, "Whoa!" Once again I almost nutted. I pulled back and kind of walked away for a second from it, you know, tried to calm myself down, like I was told to.

Pretty much what my brother told me was "Shit, man, take a sandwich or a Twinkie down there. If you're gonna bust, roll over and take a bite of Twinkie or something. Give your guy a chance to calm down." Anyway so I back up off it and walk away for a second. I settle myself and I come back. I get to rubbing on her again and I was like, "Wow, hold that open." I'm so erect and I get the head in and she starts draining on me again.

We get back on the grind and I'm moving back and forth, you know, and in the meanwhile she's pretty much got her nails all in my shoulders and I'm like, "Arghhh," about to go down cause my back's hurting. She's getting a little loud and I'm trying to jam it in there and she's pretty much like, "Stop, stop, stop." I get scared, I stop like, "Why? It's supposed to be feeling good, right?" She's kind of holding herself like, "I don't know... I want to quit." So you know, wow. Did I hurt her or something? But of course I'm a male so I'm also thinking, "Give me more."

She's kind of crying a little bit and I'm like, "Whoa, should I cry too?" I'm kind of freaked out. We get to talking and I'm like, "Wow. I'm sorry if it hurt," things like that. Anyway she's, "Oh, it's OK. It's just me."

We ease back into it and we're kissing and rubbing and I'm on top of her, she's on the bottom. I got her legs open and had her hold it open once again and I got the tip in and we're trying. She's just like, "Just be careful and be slow." So I'm being careful and slow and it's wet and it's starting to get in there a little bit. In the meanwhile I'm like getting ready to nut so I'm trying to stop and just hold it there and she's squirming and I'm like, "Whoa, easy." I'm trying to hold her from moving to calm down a little bit, all of it wasn't in yet. I'm like, "Wow, before I nut I need to at least try to get it all the way in there." Like my brother said, take your time getting in there and then when you do, take your time when you're in there.

(...and how not to)

So I'm in there, I'm getting it, I'm going, I'm going, I'm going. I quit for a minute and calm down. Got back up in there, kind of a little harder this time. It got wet again so I'm in, going and going... *boom*, she's really screaming so I kind of put my hand over her mouth a little bit and she's like, "No, no, no." And I'm like, "No, no, no what? Should I stop?" She wants me to keep going and I'm like, "But I got parents upstairs." So she grabbed a pillow and kind of covered her face with it and said, "Just do it. Just go." So I'm riding and riding and going and going and she's getting worked up and she's sweating and I'm drenched with sweat. I'm working so hard and I'm going and thirty minutes later, you know she's, "Ohhhhh!" And I'm like, "Whoa." And she says, "I'm feeling something I've never felt before." And I felt her body shake real hard and she was clenching me like I must be hurting her or something. 'Cause we were kids, we don't know anything about orgasm, climax. But we both released, it felt good. She screamed from underneath the pillow. She enjoyed herself, I enjoyed myself. I busted a nut. She busted her nut and climaxed. We're 13 years old, so our minds are blown.

Anyway we kissed and this was about 7 o'clock in the evening, streetlights go on, time for friends to go home. Time to get off the streets and get in the house, so I see her off to her place. My brothers were like, "Naw you already lost your virginity." But it was different when we both busted a nut together. That's when I look at it as like, "OK. Good, I lost my virginity. She lost hers too."

> He had great hands. The best thing is when guys know how to use their hands, and when they know how to use their mouths, it's amazing. Not so much where they use their mouth, it's how they kiss. It's not all tongue or all lip. It's like a combination of both and it like, turns you on even more. He was really sweet about it.
>
> *Becky, 23*
> *Tarzana, California*

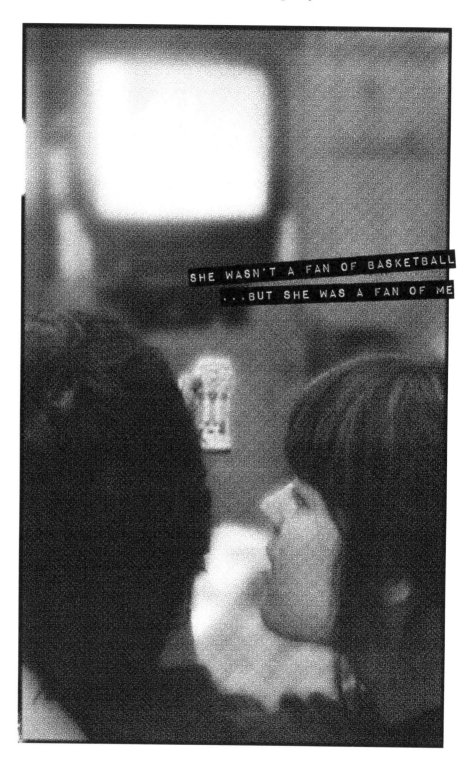

(...and how not to)

"IT'S NOT THAT BAD. IF IT WAS, EVERYONE WOULDN'T BE DOING IT."

4

This chapter title is taken from a quote in the movie, *Little Darlings* (1980), which is alluded to in a story in this chapter

    I was struck by the number of people who told me that the first time doesn't matter. That it was something you got through and you just moved on. Is this an attitude people are born with? Is it acquired from their environment? Or is it a viewpoint that develops in hindsight as a response to their own disappointing loss of virginity experience?

    A recent study by Dana Haynie and Stacy Armour from Ohio State that appears in the March 2008 issue of the *Journal of Youth and Adolescence* shows that the average age teenagers in the United States lose their virginity is 16, below the age of consent for most states. Most parents, I'm certain, would agree that men and women begin having sex much younger than they should. And perhaps this blasé, "it's no big deal", stance that people hold is a result of beginning too young, not looking before you leap, doing it before you are ready - type of experiences.

    And there's nothing inherently wrong with seeing virginity as something to get over with. You have to have that initial time to get the subsequent times which usually get increasingly enjoyable and fulfilling as time goes on. But if one could choose, who wouldn't rather have a fond memory? The following people, on the other hand, got it over with and moved on.

A VERY SPECIAL EPISODE OF "WILL & GRACE"
Heather, 34

I was in college and I had been holding out for so long so that's why I had to do it with a gay guy. It's not like I set out to have sex with a gay guy, but I was in the theatre department and gay guys were all over the place. I was just so sick of being a virgin. I was 19 and everyone else was laid by then so it was time to get it done.

Me and the gay guy were good friends and I don't know how far he had gone with other guys but we were both hetero-virgins. I didn't want to deal with the high expectations of losing it to a boyfriend and having it suck. It's the first time so it's going to be awkward anyway and it's not going to be good no matter who you're with.

He was a virgin, I was a virgin. It was the middle of the day and we were in my dorm room so we were like, "Hey, let's do it." It was more hilarious than anything else. We were laughing our asses off, especially because he was gay. But there was no equipment problem so maybe he was bi.

A year later we ended up living together. I was on him a bit, I wanted to do it again but he was like, "No." By then he was full-fledged gay. Maybe his experimental days were over, or maybe our relationship was weird by the time we lived together. Who knows? I've yet to meet anyone else who's had that experience. In fact I just told someone about it the other day and she was like, "Why didn't you do it with your high school boyfriend?" I didn't really have a high school boyfriend.

> He wanted to tittie-fuck, which I had no idea what that was but after he explained it I thought it was the dumbest thing ever. But we did it and it was not enjoyable and the whole time it was happening I was thinking, "This sucks, but I can't wait to talk about it." So I just told him, "Why don't you just put it inside of me?"
>
> *Taren, 23*
> *New York, New York*

DON'T BE SUCH A PUSSY
Lucia, 22

I'm from Mill's Landing, North Carolina. My boyfriend drove me home from school and my mother was at work so he kept pressuring me and pressuring me to do it. I didn't want to but, whatever. We did it in my mom's bed because she was away and because there wasn't enough room in my twin bed.

I was disappointed with it and after we were done he cried because he felt bad for making me do something I didn't want to do. I told him to get the hell out and come back when he could be a man. Sure I didn't want to have sex, but I wasn't going to cry about it.

(...and how not to)

SHE WASN'T A BASKETBALL FAN, BUT SHE WAS A FAN OF ME
Lance, 31

The Knicks were playing The Heat in the 1997 playoffs. It's a best of seven game series, the first team to win four games advances. The Knicks won three of the first four games, they're up 3-1. You'd think they got it made. I'm a big Knicks fan. Big, big Knicks fan. I've had season tickets the last ten years. It's all but clinched, then at the end of game five there was a big fight and half of the Knicks team gets suspended for the rest of the series.

The night I lost my virginity was the night the Knicks lost game seven of that series and wasted their chances at a championship. Tim Hardaway was killing us, bombing three-pointers from all over the floor. It was difficult to watch.

I was watching the game over at my girl's house. And it had been leading up to sex for quite some time and it was obvious by halftime that the game was over, they were getting beat so bad. I was crushed just watching these threes get drained. I don't think she could tell I was kind of catching the game during the sex, but she was on cloud nine.

LAKE SUCCESS
Jenna, 31

I was three days shy of 16. Didn't have my license yet but I was already driving around the red Subaru my sister and I were supposed to share. I was totally in love with Roy McIntyre. He was the one and only mysterious, artsy guy in our whole entire little rural town. His mom was an alcoholic so this other family that grew their own pot and like, cured their own cancer with holistic medicine felt bad for him and took him in. They let him live in the tree house in their backyard. I picked him up from his tree house and drove up to Lake Success.

We did it and I bled on the front seat. That was the most memorable moment since it wasn't that pleasurable. Although I was totally into it because I thought I was in love. And he was all into it because I was a virgin.

> Sex is amazing but you should save it for somebody you love or care about the first time, the last time, whatever time you do it cause it's going to be with you forever.
>
> *Katie, 27*
> *Denver, Colorado*

TRASH + TRASHETTE 4 EVER
Darcy, 28

It was my sophomore year and I had just turned 21. I was hanging out in Brenham, Texas, near College Station where I went to school. Brenham was in the middle of nowhere, pretty much the only thing there is to do is drink beer in a field and I was at this house party with a bunch of bull riders - pro bull riders but on the low-level circuit.

There were these twin, black bull riders named Tom and Tim. A friend of theirs was a local volunteer fire department guy nicknamed Trash. I later found out his real name was Ernie. It's so bad, I don't even remember his last name. Trash started talking to me and I thought, "Wow, he's really cute." This was already after a lot of beer; any more and he probably would have looked like Brad Pitt.

I had previously vowed to save myself for marriage, but at that point I was like, "You know what? Fuck it. I'm in college. He's hot. I'm getting hot. Why not?" He led me to this shanty back behind the house that had a mattress in it and a single, swinging flashbulb that cast creepy shadows. He found a sheet, dusted it off, and placed it over the mattress.

He thinks he's all Rico Suave and he starts giving me all these lines, "Yeah, baby. You're so beautiful." We end up doing it and it was painful. He thought I was enjoying it because I was screaming but I was actually screaming in pain. So the more I screamed, "Oh, God," he kept going harder and faster. Seeing him was kind of a shock 'cause from pictures and things you think it's supposed to look a certain way, but he was misshapen. It was curved to the right although I'm sure the funky shadows from the single light bulb didn't help how it looked.

Afterwards everyone outside the shanty was laughing their asses off. To this day all my friends from college call me Trashette. I never saw the guy again.

I was very drunk and it opened up Pandora's Box of me having sex more frequently. Once you have it, you want it more. Losing your virginity is like a gateway drug to more sex.

> I thought I was special and then at a party a co-worker was like, "Oh, I slept with him." I was like, "Really?" Then this other girl was like, "Yeah, me too." Later I found out that he had sex with almost every girl in that office.
>
> *Rhonda, 26*
> *New York, New York*

(...and how not to)

POPSICLES AND COTTON CANDY
Mandy, 18

I grew up pretty tight with my cousins and I was always the youngest. They all follow the Insane Clown Posse and I went with them every weekend to Juggalo barbecues. A Juggalo barbecue is just smoking, drinking, grubbing with a bunch of other ICP fans. Everyone paints their face and braids their hair and bumps music from their cars. Just white trash kids hanging out, something to do on a Sunday.

There was this boy there about my age. Everyone was like, "You should hook up with this kid, Garrett. He's really cool." It was not like they forced it to happen but everyone pretty much expected one day we would. And one day we did. We had our faces painted like Violent J and Shaggy 2 Dope, which was pretty cool. We were drunk, had sex in the woods, and I never talked to him again.

I stopped hanging out with my cousins after that. I stopped drinking and stuff, got away from those kind of people.

> I wasn't waiting for some magical moment. I mean, you're putting something in your crotch and making it bleed. There's no magic there.
>
> *Amy, 22*
> *Brooklyn, Ohio*

TAKE HOME SEX ED. TEST
Molly, 25

It was my freshman year of high school. My boyfriend, Patrick and I had phys. ed. together and so when exams came, since there wasn't a P.E. exam we all got three hours off in the middle of the day. We decided that since we didn't have anything to do that we would catch a ride with some seniors to his house.

This had all been planned out. I was 14, I didn't have anything sexy so I stole some black underwear and a matching pretty bra from my mom's underwear drawer. Patrick was always badgering me about it and I "loved him" so I was going to do it. And once the wheels were in motion, once we were on our way in the back of the seniors' truck, and once we were in his room on the top bunk next to the ceiling it's not like you can say, "Oh, never mind. I'm uncomfortable." I almost said no, but once your pants come off you can't just back out of it. I mean the poor guy had been trying for six months. He makes this whole elaborate plan, and he didn't have a house key because he was only 15 years old so he had a secret key made to get us in – all so the parents couldn't find out. You're at his house, you're in his bunk bed… you gotta do it.

Afterwards we walked to the mall, met back up with the seniors, caught a ride back to the school and made the bus ride home. His whole plan worked without a hitch. It wasn't fun but I'm glad I got it over with. We were a 14 and 15-year-old in love, but how in love really are you? You're just so dumb at 14.

And it hurt to walk back to the mall.

DO ALL LESBIANS GO THROUGH THIS?
Kara, 27

The first girl I ever dated or slept with was a girl I met my freshman year of college. I went to my first year of college in Southeastern Kentucky and I met her through some mutual friends. We had an algebra class together. Because I went to church, I was like the "good girl." I never really had huge crushes on girls but just some slight curiosity. I dated guys but it was a take it or leave it kind of a thing. And I grew up in the bible belt, Southeastern Kentucky, where there were all of maybe five gay people in the area and everybody knew who they were. I actually ended up hanging out with the gay people even before I came out and it got around to my church director, everybody knew everybody's business down there, and he was like, "If you believe homosexuality is OK then you don't belong here."

Anyway she was in my algebra class in college. We never talked except, "Hey do you have a pencil?" or asking the answer to a question or something like that. But I was introduced to her through the theater group I was in and one of her friends was in theater and we finally met at a party and she totally stalked me at the party. I was freaking out about it because my first thought was that I didn't want my mom to find out I was a lesbian. But she was pretty persistent. She was incredibly forward. But not pushy, not like disgusting. A lot of gay people get a bad rap that they're horribly pushy and they want to convert everybody, but it wasn't like that. She was answering questions for me that I didn't know I was asking.

It was a very educational experience. Not just physically but sort of sexuality-wise. It was new to me, and yet I knew it was everything I wanted to pursue. So I actually lost my girl virginity to her in her parents' bed. I think we went out to the movies or something like that, hanging out. But we had to hang out in another town over because if anybody had seen us and knew us then it would get around and I wasn't ready for that.

We went back to her parents' house and... it was one of the most awkward, eye-opening experiences of probably my entire life. I'm a bit of a tease anyway so I'd been teasing her about getting physical but would never let her do anything to me because even though I wanted her to do things to me, I didn't want to let her because then it would mean I'm gay. It took me awhile until I was ready to make that leap

It had been a couple months, at least. Probably three, four months since we met at the party. And I mean, we hung out a lot too and she actually ended up tutoring me in algebra because I sucked. She kind of took that whole teacher aspect with me, somebody who was older and more experienced. She was a lesbian in high school. She was one of the "known" lesbians in town. She was a dyke straight from the womb.

Basically it was from then on that I knew that, you know, I didn't want to be with guys anymore. It was so much better than my first time with a guy, and I'm sure that every lesbian says that... but it really was. I don't even know how to explain it. It probably wasn't even that good of sex. It's not as good as the sex I'm having now but we all learn.

She was very kind and understanding, which helped since I was so shy and afraid. And she didn't ask anything of me. You know, she was just like, "Relax, lay back, let me do this to you. Let me make you feel good," and she did and obviously I'm glad I did it because I live that lifestyle now.

(...and how not to)

TO WANK OR TO SHAG? THAT IS THE QUESTION
George, 34

I met her in high school, grade 11, during a play we were doing, *The Miracle Worker*, the touching story of Helen Keller. I had a minor part: I was the younger brother. I had a crush on this girl playing Annie Sullivan, the miracle worker herself.

She was a terrible actress; it was a terrible production really. But Madge and I went out for... I don't know, it seemed like forever and an eternity. But as you know, in grade 11 every day lasted an eternity. We broke up several times over various ridiculous 16-year-old problems we had at the time. We hadn't slept together although we'd done everything else up to that point.

We went through our last major bust-up and although we weren't dating we were still in contact and we decided we both wanted to lose our virginity with each other. The night we agreed upon she was somebody else's prom date from another high school. I've often wondered about him, you know it's prom night and I'm sure he was fully expecting to get it on. But she went to the prom with the guy and after the dance she changed out of her dress and snuck in through my bedroom window.

If I remember correctly (and there's no reason to assume that I do), I asked her to wear my favorite sweater of hers and she did, in fact, climb in through my window wearing that very sweater. We knew this was what we were going to do and we had to be quiet because my parents were around, asleep, but even so we had to be quiet.

There was the pageantry and drama of me putting on a condom for the first time. And of course the important thing for me was what music was playing. I had spent quite a bit of time ruminating about what tape I wanted in my tape player and I decided it would be best to lose my virginity to The Beatles' *Abbey Road*. We started with side one and I actually interrupted the action at one point to flip the tape over so actual penetration occurred somewhere on side two.

Compared to the acts we'd done before, the sex itself was a bit disappointing. I only realized many years later that sex could be a lot better other than the very standard sort of missionary deal, which was all we tried. I guess 'cause we talked about it so much or we had done so much before it was just a regular orgasm. Then she cried a little bit and I tried to comfort her. I asked, "What's wrong?" She said, "Well I don't know... we had sex, I'm not a virgin anymore." And I said, "Yeah, that's a good thing. I don't feel like crying."

Around that time I was reading a book, sort of a biography about John Lennon by his childhood best friend. When John Lennon lost his virginity before the best friend did, he met the best friend the next day and Lennon told him, "Yeah got my first fuck," and the friend says, "Yeah how was it?" Lennon said, "Well, actually... I'd rather have a wank." So the next day I met up with my best friend and I was all ready to use this and I just said, "So yeah. I had my first fuck last night." He said, "Well?" I said, "Rather have a wank." He said, "Hmm. OK."

Later things went right in the toilet and I think she probably regrets that her first was with me, which I regret that she regrets. But I was glad I did it and I was glad I did it with Madge because I did really like her and we had been together for awhile.

THE OTHER WOMAN
Lynette, 23

I was 15, Ben was 16. We had been friends for about six months and the whole time I knew him, he was dating this other girl. He had been dating this other girl for about two years and it never happened between them, I have no idea why.

We started messing around and one night I snuck out of my mom's house and got a ride from a friend over to his place. I snuck into his house and it happened, first time for both of us. I was the other woman, which made me feel daring. I spent the night there and when he woke up early the next morning to do his paper route I went to go hide out in his basement until he got back but his dad caught me. So Ben made up a story about how my mom was out of town and I was supposed to stay the night at a friend's house but her and I got into a fight so that's why I was there. It was quick thinking on his part.

We continued seeing each other on the sly and then he went crazy and tried to kill himself at school because he found out his girlfriend was seeing another guy and he just flipped out. Like it was OK for him to see someone else, but not her. It was more of a cry for help than anything. He cut his stomach with a six-inch knife in the hallway with tons of people around. He had these three really huge cuts across his stomach and he got put in the psych ward for a week. I didn't go to school the whole time he was in the hospital because the whole thing was just too much to handle.

I don't regret my first. It happened. I just didn't care, I mean... shit happens to people.

THE LESSER OF TWO EVILS
Vera, 19

It was with this guy I had been dating for just a couple months. I don't know, I guess it's what every girl wants or thinks they want. I was older, 19, because I was the "wait for marriage" girl. Then I realized I have a little problem with commitment and decided I didn't want to get married and thought, "Well shit. I can't go my whole life and not ever fuck anyone."

Me and this guy had been dating for a couple of months and he was obviously more experienced than I was so one night at like three o'clock in the morning we were in my room watching of all things a fucking Frank Lloyd Wright documentary on The Learning Channel. Not the sexiest thing to get you in the mood but boredom can get you in the mood too.

I couldn't tell him I loved him and I guess that sex was easier. I didn't want to say it and lie, so sex was just an easy way to sidestep the whole love issue like, "All right, well... how about this?" He was like, "I love you. I love you," and I couldn't say that part so... let me just give you what else you want so you can forget about the love part. That's what every girl wants, right, to be in love? But if you're not you still at least want someone who... you know... likes you.

We went on the couch, and then on the floor, it was like, "Let's just do it." It wasn't a minute and a half or two-minute long story because, yeah it was good. He knew exactly what he was doing.

(...and how not to)

LIFE IMITATES ART
Joanie, 40

You have to understand the movie *Little Darlings*. The two girls in the movie made a bet to see who was going to lose their virginity first. The good girl makes it all up, lies and says she does it when really she doesn't. And the naughty, fun girl does it but feels guilty and says she didn't do it. Anyway my friend and I made a *Little Darlings* type of bet. This was in 1981, I was 15.

In Colorado Springs there's a military base so there's always a lot of army guys around. My friend and I used to hang out at the roller skating rink and one night we hooked up with these GI's, these 19 or 20-year-old guys hanging out at the roller rink looking to pick up girls... looking to pick up my dumb ass.

I decided I was going to go for it and it was really awful. We went back to my house and we did it on my mother's waterbed. Really, it was awful. I was freaked out about being in my mom's bed; it hurt, and I had given no thought to the possibility of messing up the sheets, which of course we did. I was like, "Oh my god. We got to clean the sheets." He was older; you'd think he'd know about all that stuff.

I didn't tell my best friend about it for a while, just like in the movie. She said she made it with his buddy, the other Army guy, in the backseat of the car. But she was full of shit and I later found out she was not telling the truth, also just like in the movie.

How to Lose Your Virginity

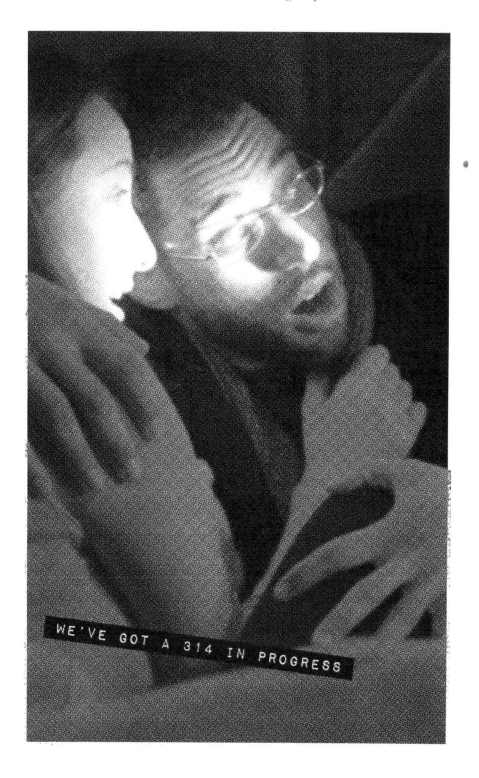

(...and how not to)

"WHAT'S GOING ON IN THERE?!"

5

There's an illicit quality to young love. The prospect of getting found out by the parents, the cops, or even friends is inseparable from the thought of many on the verge of doing it. And not just getting caught but, as in the case of Carolina in "THIS ONE TIME... IN THE BAND ROOM", getting found out. "Can they tell?" "Will they know?" That fear alone is enough for some to postpone their loss of virginity.

Now some people revel in getting caught, fantasize about it. While I didn't find anyone who purposefully engineered a first time where they can get walked in on, the act of getting caught affected people differently. For some they were mortified, for others it lightened the mood.

YOU'RE BETTER THAN PATRICK, EVERYONE THINKS SO
Charlie, 30

My friends and I decided to go to a party at some guy's house instead of to our high school football game. There was about eight of us, guys and girls. One of the girls was my close friend Patrick's ex-girlfriend who took his virginity.

The house we were partying at, some of the dirtiest humans in the world lived there. They were your typical hillbillies: cars on blocks in the front yard, the dad was a Civil War reenactor. The oldest brother was a divorced, out-of-work mechanic who actually lived inside a car that was parked on the side of the house. His father wouldn't let him stay in the house, so he stayed in the car. The guy we knew from this family sold drugs at the high school. We used to go over there to huff gas 'cause his dad didn't care if we huffed gas. This is the kind of house it was.

Throughout the course of the evening, we were drinking and playing drinking games and Patrick's ex-girlfriend was flirting with me. I'm 16 and up to this point I had never kissed a girl. I had never done anything. I had never had a girlfriend in my life, anything, nothing. I'm totally a clean slate. The night wanders on, we're flirting around. I flung some bottle caps down her top. She was very big chested and this move apparently worked 'cause we eventually took it to our drug dealer friend's bedroom.

His bed was stacked with dirty clothes. There's car parts – literally car parts in his room, stuff he was working on. So we basically heaped onto this bed, on top of his filthy laundry. It was disgusting were if not for the fact I was about to get laid.

We start getting into it. I had the condom on and I was like raring to go. I hadn't even got inside her yet, hadn't even got her pants off and she starts saying things to me like, "Oh you're so much better than Patrick." They had just slept together like the week before. So I'm like, "Ok, I guess then if you say so. I am? Well then I am." Then I hear these falsetto voices mocking her through the window next to the bed, "Oh Charlie, you're so much better than Patrick!"

So I'm trying to keep going, trying to concentrate. I think I'm getting into it right. I think I have a rhythm built up. Then the door opens up and I sort of comically put my hand over my hip to cover her and myself thinking that was enough guard, like no one would see us. She's like, "Oh, don't stop. Don't stop." The guy's like, "Don't worry about me." He picks up some car parts and leaves.

We proceed to have sex as best as I knew how, finished, and laid there for awhile I guess to make it more meaningful. We got up, we went back out into the party and everybody was kind of laughing and almost cheering. So she obviously didn't care. I dated her for a month after that and we had sex three more times.

I made the mistake of getting in an argument with someone in the cafeteria about getting laid and I said, "Well we've had sex four times." So somebody wrote on the wall in the guys bathroom, "Watch out for Charlie Felloni, he's fucked four times." I didn't live that down for about a year.

(...and how not to)

THIS ONE TIME... IN THE BAND ROOM
Carolina, 21

OK – beginning of my freshman year in high school. She was a senior and we were in band together. It was after a football game in the band hall, in a cubby hole where a big instrument is supposed to go. It was around midnight and we were in school with nobody around. It was possible we could get caught so it took us awhile to get working up to where we just couldn't stop and there was no turning back.

This was after the last football game of the year so everybody stayed on the field and everything and we kind of cut out early 'cause we had planned to go to this party elsewhere or whatever. Then we ended up not leaving and staying at the band hall. It was quite awhile before anybody else came in so there wasn't really a chance of anyone walking in on us, but regardless there was that exciting intensity of the possibility of someone walking in on us.

I was a lesbian. She was bi-curious and single at the time. Conversations and her curiosity kind of led us down that path, with me mostly leading the way. It was one of those things that, ironically enough, I mean they made a movie with a joke about it but we ended up using a musical instrument – hers, a flute. I played clarinet but the flute was a little more manageable.

As it turned out there was a video camera installed right above us so all you saw on the video was feet sticking out of a cubby hole. And nobody could really say what was happening but it was kind of obvious. Thus, even though no one walked in on us, we still got found out.

The band instructor confronted me personally because I was actually freshmen band president. Pretty funny but at the time real embarrassing. They took me into an office and showed me the videotape and asked me to explain and I started crying. I mean it was emotional because it was the first time with any kind of person, first... exposure. Nobody had ever seen my body before ever, ever. Then she did. So it was intense in a good way but incredibly embarrassing afterwards to the point where after the relationship I remained celibate for awhile.

Eventually it got out and people knew about it and we both had to quit band. And it escalated from there.

When rumors started to spread we were badgered by other students. This was in middle of nowhere Pflugerville, Texas, so of course we felt the brunt of conservative prejudice. We got cornered by a bunch of football players and it got so bad that she ended up moving away. When she moved the relationship ended. I tried to join band again after she left but they still deemed my presence as inappropriate and wouldn't let me.

As the years progressed and I got older I ended up exploring different venues and going into the opposite gender but that first physical experience, that's pretty much the highest rated ever because of the intensity of getting caught. Doing something bad in a bad place makes it that much better.

If I left anything out, it's pretty much just the hardcore details.

WE'VE GOT A 314 IN PROGRESS
Samantha, 24

When I was 14 and my boyfriend was 16 I banged him in the backseat of his car in the parking lot of a cemetery in Olmsted Falls. Then a cop showed up right in the middle of it, that really sucked, and I got arrested for indecent exposure.

I had to call my folks, it was their anniversary and they were at a party at someone else's house. That was just great. So I had to call and interrupt their party to tell them I was arrested. They were pissed, they had to come pick me up, and the next day my mom gave me a handful of condoms.

I was grounded for a few weeks and I couldn't see any of my friends or my boyfriend. And I had to go to court for indecent exposure, but the cop didn't show up so I got off with no charges.

TANGERINE
Farrah, 21

I met Bradley where I'm from in Northeast Philadelphia when I was 11 or 12 years old. We met outside of a restaurant called 'Wings To Go' and I thought he was cute so I started talking to him because I'm kind of an aggressive person that way. I did date his best friend first but then we got together and after our first kiss and ended up dating for six years.

He was a long-haired guitar player who I later molded into a musician, so to speak. I introduced him to The Beatles, Zeppelin, The Who, and all that good stuff. We were loving hippies trying to change the world – all about peace. He's a good person but to this day he's still very young and immature.

I wanted to wait to have sex until after high school for some reason. Basically hold on to it as long as I could. Not to be cool or different, just to feel good about myself that I was able to keep it for so long. I was just kissing when so many of my friends, who are now in their 20s and have three-year-olds, were already having sex. And I wasn't expecting to marry the man but I at least wanted him to be someone special and that's exactly what my long-haired guitar player was to me. He was special and he loved my family and my family loved him and we had a good relationship so I waited all four years of high school until the day before I graduated.

I didn't let him know until he was right in my room. I had candles all over and I always wanted to lose it to Led Zeppelin, my favorite band ever. So I had *Led Zeppelin III* on and that album has that great song, "Since I've Been Loving You," which is an appropriate song to lose it to because it's kind of like this guy going over this girl's house to bang her. She's got a man but this is her back-door man. We got this sexy song, we got the candles all lit, it's the day before graduation and just as we're about to get started my older sister walks in and turns on all the lights.

(...and how not to)

For most people it probably would have taken them away from it but for me it made me more into it because I simply started laughing, then he started laughing and it kind of like broke the ice. So it was kind of like a good thing my sister walked in on us. My older sister has always been kind of protective of me but she was proud that I held my virginity for as long as I did because she had given hers away so easy.

My first time was very, very, very magical and touching and beautiful and... kind of everything that I hoped it would be but never thought it would because I had heard so many negative things about it. We continued to see each other for another three years after that, which is good.

Of course it was painful and all that good stuff, but I knew that I was in somebody's arms who loved me and who I loved back 100%. It was like I was in heaven, complete heaven. It was one of the best things that ever happened to me. It opened many doors to see the world in a different way, to see what else is out there.

The day after graduation, my best friend noticed the change in me. She was like, "You had sex didn't you?" I was like, "Really? How did you know?" And she said, "I could just tell. You're glowing."

My generation is very different. We're, I would say, very easy. Very, very easy. For me it was special. I was the only one out of anybody I knew who was still a virgin. I took total pride in it. And now I take pride in being a non-virgin.

About a year and a half after it happened, I was out with my parents and my grandmother, we were out having lunch on a Sunday afternoon and out of the blue mom says, "Oh, I talked to Connie, Rita's mom. Rita's pregnant." My first thought was, "Oh my God." I sat there for about 10 minutes before it dawned on me... it's been a year and a half. It can't be mine. But for about 10 minutes I really thought, "OK. I'm 14... either they'll kill me or they're going to make us get married in Arkansas." That was a heart-stopping moment.

Lenny, 40
Austin, Texas

AS GOOD A PLACE AS ANY
Daniel, 28

It started in summer camp after 11th grade, a Jewish summer camp, while we were taking a bus trip from Michigan up to Alaska. It took us a week and a half getting there, we spent four weeks in Alaska, and then a week driving back. The second night of traveling we were camping somewhere in Calgary and I ended up making out with this girl I met on the trip. Didn't really think anything of it. Went through the rest of the trip and made out with a couple of the other girls. When we got back to Michigan, that first girl I made out with introduced me to her friend, this Goth chick, Celia, who was really intriguing because I was like this good suburban boy looking for trouble but every girl I was in camp with was from the same typical kind of Michigan Jewish American Princess crowd. This Goth girl was anything but.

One day I heard her on the phone arguing with her mom telling her she's a fucking bitch and telling her to fuck off and all this stuff and I was just like, "Wow. This girl is really cool." I had always got along with my family so it was alluring to see someone rebelling.

One night we were hanging out at my camp counselor's apartment. She went to school at Michigan State University, which is right near where I grew up. She was probably six or seven years older than us and we were hanging out there and it was this counselor's 24th birthday party and she and all of her friends went to the bar and left us there to meet up with them later. So the Goth chick and I went into the bedroom and we started making out.

Anyway I dug around in her drawer and found a condom and we were making out and I ended up like having sex on the counselor's bed. You know it was like probably 25-30 seconds of glory for me. Afterwards we shared a cigarette and we talked about how I was pretty brief.

We drove to the bar and we were like hanging out with the counselor and all of her friends and they were buying us beer and we were like, "Sweet. We're underage and we're drinking." The next day I got a call from the counselor and she was just like, "I can't fucking believe you did that. That is so rude," and all that stuff. And I was like, "What are you talking about?" And she was like, "I found your fucking condom on the floor next to the bed." I was in such a post-sex haze that I forgot to clean up after ourselves.

I went out with the Goth girl for about a year and then she started doing heroin and left me for another woman. I still think about her to this day. The counselor and I worked it out and made up. We smoked a bunch of pot and I apologized.

(...and how not to)

UNWELCOME GUEST
Vivian, 25

I was visiting my sister in Virginia Beach for an extended stay. She was in the Navy and lived with her boyfriend and a married couple. The wife of the married couple went out of town for the weekend. Me and her husband got a little intoxicated and had sex. It just happened. You go upstairs together and you walk into the same room and you take off your clothes and you get down and dirty. But we had been putting out signals to each other since I first got there.

His wife came back the next day. They got into some argument so he told her that we slept together. She didn't believe him so he showed her the condom and she flipped out. She came after me and we got into this big fight. I punched her, busted her lip, she fell over. She apologized to me the next day.

I didn't feel bad they were married. That's all on him. I had a good time. It was fabulous.

GRANDMA'S HOME
Gavin, 24

In my hometown in Michigan I felt pressured to lose my virginity somewhere between the ages of 12 and 14. There was a lot of pressure to be down and how you be down is you bang a girl. I had a girl who felt that pressure too. The pressure was on us. We talked about it for awhile and I was wanting to experiment so we skipped school one day and I went over to her house. The problem was that her grandmother was upstairs.

We're down on her couch and it took maybe five minutes of working it. I was like, "Maybe it's this hole. This one is tight. OK. I think?" After five minutes of trying, I got in there and it felt great. I didn't wear a condom. Condom?! At 13, I didn't give a shit about a condom.

After I was in there we went on for about five to seven good minutes. It was almost like a "hood" sin to touch your own dick, so I had no previous knowledge. Didn't know how it was going to end. I was going. I was shaking and gyrating and everything and then I just exploded all over their black leather couch. Just all over it.

We were cleaning everything up and her grandmother came downstairs and she had to know there was sex in the air because she was like, "Just get out. Get out. Get out, boy. I don't know who you are. Get out!" I ran out of the house with my pants are halfway down and tripped down the porch steps. I pulled up my pants and ran the rest of the way home.

CRIME SCENE INVESTIGATOR
Nancy, 39

I was about to turn 16 and I really loved Joshua and he loved me. We lived in nearby neighborhoods and had mutual friends so we kept on encountering each other. But we never really actually became attracted to each other until three or four months before we did the deed. My mom didn't really approve of him, therefore I thought he must be OK. That and he was really hot.

The first time was in the backseat of his mom's Cadillac. But I actually lost my virginity twice. It took two times before it actually went away completely. We used a sock to wipe up all the mess the second time and his friend found the sock lying on the floor in his room. That's how everybody found out that he and I were more than just friends.

> The weird thing was that while I lost my virginity, his sister was sleeping next to us in bed. It's hard to believe she could be sleeping the whole time.
>
> *Alexis, 30*
> *Gent, Belgium*

I KNOW THAT GIRL!
Eduardo, 22

I was 17, the girl was 15 and she was a slut. My friends knew her and they were all, "She likes you." I was like, "Oh. All right." You know I was 17, the funny little bastard I was, I went up to her and was like, "Wha... uh... yeah, um... wah, wah, wah..." Somehow I got her phone number and she got mine.

My parents were gone for a long weekend and she called. She came over. I was 17 and didn't know what to do. She was 15, but knew exactly what to do. Definitely not her first time. Definitely, definitely not her first time, which was kind of creepy yet kind of good at the same time.

It's three o'clock in the afternoon and we're in my room. My sister gets home from school and barges in my room like always, saw us and screamed, "That girl's in my third period geometry class." It was no good. I got laid but my sister got a story about her older brother. Lock your doors, that's all I've got to say. Lock your doors.

(...and how not to)

DISTURBIA
Charlie, 33

I ran on the cross-country team in high school. There was a big bunch of us who started training really early in the summer. We were running miles and miles every day so we got to be this big kind of tight-knit group. That's how I sort of fell in love with this girl named Karen on the cross-country team.

It was one of those typical teen movie scenarios where my parents were out of town and she comes over because she knows I'm alone. That was it – we had sex. The only remarkable thing about it was that I bought these lubricated Trojan condoms. And when I put it on and it was all wet and she got pissed off at me because she thought I had cum already. I had to convince her, "No, no. That's not cum. It's the lube on the condom."

What made it *the worst* teen movie scenario possible was apparently I didn't have my blinds shut all the way. A few hours after it happened this neighbor kid from across the street called me up like, "Charlie?" And I was like, "*Yeahhh?* What's up?" And he said, "Charlie? Uh..." He didn't really say anything and I was like, "Yeah. What's going on?" He's like, "Uh... um... is everything OK over there?" I was like, "Yeah... everything OK over there?"

Apparently he saw the whole thing happen or who knows, maybe his parents saw it happening too. But it was the worst aftermath of losing your virginity that a guy can ever have because it got back to my parents.

It was the worst, most humiliating thing having my parents sit me down on the sofa and give me the big talk. They were pissed off that I had done it while they weren't home. They were pissed off and freaked out because I was 17 and she was 15. But I had done what any red-blooded 17-year-old teenage boy would do while his parents are out of town which is fuck a girl.

My parents did everything they could to paint what had happened in the worst possible light. Telling me that if her parents found out they'd kill me, or saying I better pray she doesn't miss her period. It was the worst way they could have dealt with it... ever. It was terrible.

The having the sex part, that was great. And she and I got together and did it a few times after that. But the whole aftermath with my parents was, I thought, inexcusable. And my parents are great parents, but I always sort of held that incident against them. They could've been a whole lot cooler about it.

> I've never seen a human move faster than my girlfriend – pulling everything with her – the covers, the pillows, everything to the corner of my bed and leaving me naked wearing a condom, looking at my brother who says, "Yeah man, that's all you."
>
> *Richard, 23*
> *Washington, D.C.*

WILLINGLY TRICKED INTO HER TENT
Rich, 20

I worked in a video store and my boss invited me to her graduation party. We were good friends, sort of a brother-sister kind of a thing. So I went to her party and I got really drunk, the most trashed I'd ever been at that point in my life.

My boss's younger sister was the same age as me and she was hitting on me uncontrollably. No one was allowed to leave drunk so there were all these tents set up in the backyard. I ended up sleeping with her in a tent. It was pretty shitty. While we were in there I heard her mom say, "What? There's a boy in there? Get the shotgun." I immediately ran out of the tent and passed out in some secluded corner of the backyard.

The next day I was back at the video store. We were closing up and all of a sudden my boss walks in and throws her huge ring of keys at me like fast pitch, as hard as she could. She screams her head off because not only was it with her sister but she also found out the sex was drunkenly unprotected.

She yelled for awhile saying that I could have gotten her sister pregnant and she doesn't know what I could have caught because her sister was by no means a virgin. Then her mom called me and said I had to tell my parents or she was going to tell them for me.

My dad was on the front porch smoking a cigarette when I got home. So here I am, 15 and I had to tell my conservative parents: "Listen. At that graduation party, I got drunk as fuck, stoned off my ass and then had unprotected sex with my boss' younger sister." His response was, "Well I knew this was going to happen. I just hoped that you'd use a condom. What the fuck were you thinking?" He hollered for my mother to come outside and her response was kind of like, "Oh my god! My only boy!" They grounded me for a week.

My boss and I made up. She knew I was young and drunk and she knew that her slut sister was hitting on me crazy. At first she was like, "Ohmigod, you had sex with my sister." Then she was like, "Oh my god. My sister totally duped you into having sex with her," which she kind of did... but she kind of didn't. I mean when you're so drunk that you can't even sit in a chair and some random hot girl is sticking her tongue in your ear, what are you gonna do? You're gonna do whatever she tells you to do.

You know, many people would regret something like that but honestly, I don't regret it. It's good to get it over with. I didn't really know her and if she was bored by it, well I didn't have to deal with that later. If she had been a girl that I really cared about, and she was like, "Huh? That's that?" It would have felt shitty to put someone you cared about through that.

> I wake up after it's done and she whispers in my ear, "Thank you." I fucking roll over to the side, I was 14 years old, I roll over and I look over the side of my dad's bed and there's a condom there and I fucking started crying. All my friends busted in and saw me crying.
>
> *Gary, 22*
> *West Park, Ohio*

(...and how not to)

I READ IT SO IT MUST BE TRUE
Tamara, 23

I had read in Cosmo about this study that said the average age that boys lose their virginity is 16. Average age that girls lose their virginity is 17. So I was like, "I'm 17. Time's a wastin'."

My family was about to take a trip to Florida for spring break. Being from an all-girls school there was, of course, slim pickings so I decided I was not gonna come back from Florida unless I was a woman. With that plan in mind I signed up for teen volleyball one night but it got cancelled, so I wound up wandering the beach at night in St. Petersburg, Florida.

I ran into three guys who ranged from 16, one was 17, and one was 19. The beach was pretty deserted, considering it was spring break. They were totally the first guys I saw. We started talking and they were acting like stupid guys and one of them said, "Hey, why don't you give us head?" I said, "OK." I would have managed to bring it up even if they hadn't.

I wound up leading them all over various parts of this beach. First we went to the sauna, I was like, "No, this isn't right." One of the guys like kind of pinched my stomach and said, "Oh, you have rolls on your stomach." The other guys were like, "Shut... up... dude," and, "Don't piss off the girl." Whatever, I was a woman on a mission.

We finally found this secluded place on the beach. The story I tell most people is that I met just one guy and we slept together but really I met these three guys and I went down on the first one. That took maybe 10 minutes. Then I went down on the second one, that took like almost an hour 'cause he'd been swimming, or whatever. He tried to get me to sleep with him, but I said no 'cause he was all vulgar and in my face about popping my cherry. Plus the third one was much cuter.

So I wound up sleeping with the third one and it was so cheesy. Like when we finished he threw the condom over the wall at his friends, then they threw it back and it hit us and I screamed.

That happened maybe halfway through the trip and I didn't hang out with them again because obviously I didn't have a cell phone or anything back then. But there was one time when the guy I slept with was walking into the hotel. I didn't see him at first, then all of a sudden I felt this weird jolt of electricity I turned and it was him. I thought it was good sex only because I had no basis for comparison. My legs hurt the next day. I think I pulled a groin muscle. That was the only thing that hurt. I thought I got off, but that was before I really understood what getting off was.

After we got back home my mom confronted me with, "Did you have sex in Florida?" And I was like, "Nooo... what are you talking about?" And she tried to like hedge around it, she's like, "I think you did," And I was like, "That's ridiculous." And finally she broke down and just was like, "I read your diary." She started crying. My diary was in my bag and she found it. I had been keeping it for ten years and she never read it before. She found out everything, all the explicit details.

How to Lose Your Virginity

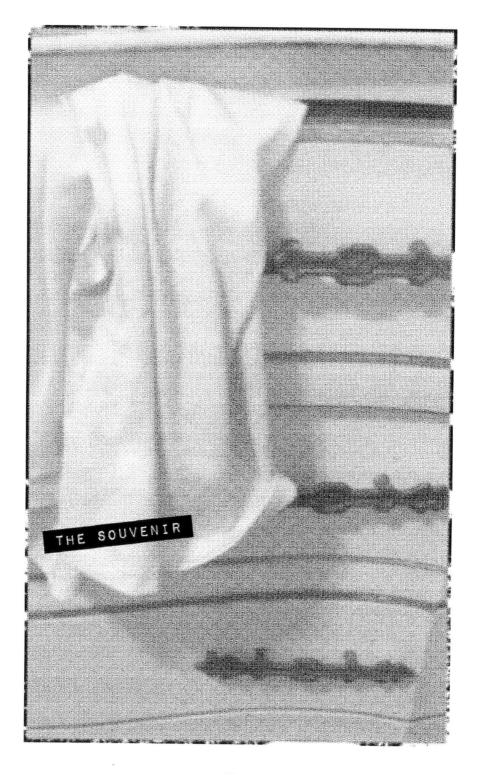

(...and how not to)

"TONIGHT IS THE NIGHT YOU MAKE ME A WOMAN / MAN"

6

I went to New Orleans for Mardi Gras the year after Hurricane Katrina hit. I found cheap fares to Austin, Texas, the drawback being that I had an 8-hour solo drive from the airport with Fat Tuesday awaiting me on the other side. As I drove east on I-10, pushing 75 mph in an effort to make good time, I heard on the radio, to me, an unfamiliar song "Tonight Is the Night" by Betty Wright. In it she sings, "Tonight is the night you make me a woman. You said you'd be gentle with me and I hope you will." An appropriate sentiment for the work I had set out for myself, and a reminder that despite some people's assumptions, not all first sexual experiences are clumsy or disappointing. There are those lucky few who do have amazing, monumental, and even joyous firsts.

These stories aren't completely devoid of clumsiness or awkwardness. Nobody gets behind the wheel of a car for the first time and automatically knows how to handle it. And, as is often the case with memories, they sometimes sweeten with age. But these entries represent the type of experience that many aspire to have, or wish they had.

SECRET RECIPE
Debra, 25

I was younger than I thought I would be when it happened, but it was with my best friend. We're still friends, have been for over 15 years. It was in my house, in my room, so I was in a place where I felt safe. But I was still all nervous and shaky. He was above me, and he started shaking too. The bed started to move. I was like, "What's the deal?" And he said the coolest thing, "It's my first time. I'm nervous too." It was great because he's a boy and boys don't say that.

Afterwards we made brownies and I didn't let them cook all the way. I just got excited and wanted the chocolate as soon as I could get it. They were hot and still gooey. Now, whenever I smell brownies it reminds me of the first time.

RIPE FOR THE PICKING
Alison, 26

I grew up in Canyon, Texas, which is 15 miles south of Amarillo. Summer was upon us and I was about to go into high school when I met this boy who had just moved with his father from Omaha, Nebraska. Wesley was really cute and really shy. He knew nobody in school and I befriended him. The last days of that school year we would walk home together.

We became close friends that whole summer. We would go Rollerblading during the day, and at night I would sneak and wait underneath his bedroom window and he had never snuck out before so I was a bad influence on him. I was never bad either, but he just gave me reason to be a bad girl. We would sneak out to this house being built and fool around; it was like the shell of a house. He was going into the eighth grade and you know, boys at that age are really awkward and stuff but he could tell, he knew I was making the moves on him.

Wesley had a strawberry garden in his backyard and one afternoon he picked and cleaned all these strawberries for me. We're outside laying in the grass, I had my head on his lap and he's feeding me these strawberries. He was wearing an unbuttoned long sleeve shirt with the sleeves rolled up and a white t-shirt underneath, real tight Levis jeans with no shoes. It was such a good… everything. He's feeding me these strawberries and I totally kiss him. Then he led me to his room. He was really cute and I wanted to deflower him, I wanted him to deflower me. He said he'd never done this before. I said, "Me neither." It just happened and it was real nice.

I had a real shaky rapport with men up to that point. My parents were divorced so I didn't really trust guys. So this was a very positive male experience and it gave me a reason to trust guys but he eventually moved back to Nebraska. His dad was like the Gestapo and wouldn't let him do anything. He felt really repressed because of it so he moved back with his mom in Omaha.

The song "Omaha" by Counting Crows always made me think of him and I've always really loved that song because of that boy.

(...and how not to)

I COULD'VE BEEN A STEP DAD
Kyle, 47

New Year's Eve. I didn't have any plans so I went to a party with Leonard, one of my older brother's friends. Her name was Suzanne. I'll save her last name for myself. Can't remember the names of the other girls that Leonard brought.

We were drinking. So she thought I was around 17, but I was really 12. I was just with older people and I looked older, big for my age. I weighed about 130 lbs. so I just looked like a skinny 17-year-old. She'd expected me to stay without having to call home and ask my mom if I could spend the night so I obliged. I remember drinking and having a good time. She was a knockout.

Suzanne and I went up to the bedroom. Leonard stayed down there with two of the girls. He got it on with both the girls downstairs. I went upstairs. Got into my thing, whatever I could do at the age of 12. Right in the middle of it all, she asks if I was gay. I had no moves, I was very innocent.

I mean, back in the '70s they didn't have all the stuff they have on TV now, or the Internet. The pornos now. They didn't have any of that shit when I was a kid. And it's a little scary and overwhelming seeing a naked body for the first time. My older brother used to have Playboy mags. So the first I got was just like, tit shots. That was as far as I had ever seen. So the whole thing was nerve-wracking.

I really do believe she thought I was 17 and assumed I'd had a couple experiences under my belt. Ended up almost going to Texas with her. She asked me if I knew how to drive. I said, "Sure, I know how to drive." I had already had sex with her, might as well keep the illusion going.

She had an eight or nine-month old child crying in the crib next to her bed, which I felt bad about. Even at that age I was like, "This is not right." She had her own place though so I figured, "OK, she knows what she's doing." She asked me if I could drive her truck to Texas with her. Split the driving, go down there and start a new life. So I was like, "Yeah, sure. Sounds pretty good."

Now the guy I went with, Leonard, the next morning he says, "Kyle, we need to cut out. We need to get you back to your house." I said, "You go. I'm staying here." He said, "Ok, if you want to stay here, suit yourself."

About three hours after Leonard left, she told me she had to go shopping for the kid. So I was there by myself with her baby. The doorbell rang, I answered it in my underwear, and it was her older brother. He was like, "Where's Suzanne?" I said, "She went out to buy her kid some baby food." Then he just kind of forced his way inside the door, sat on the couch, told me to go put my pants on. I was going up the stairs and that's when my two older brothers and Leonard knocked on the door.

I'm standing in my underwear and they ask me what the hell I was doing there. I told them "This is my new home. I'm with Suzanne now." They dragged my ass out of the house, threw me in the fucking car and beat the shit out of me the whole drive home. When we got back, my mom beat the shit out of me some more.

So that's how I lost my virginity. She was 18 or 19 and thought I was 17 and knew how to drive a truck. That was the first and the last time I saw her. Never heard what became of her.

SALUTE THE RED, WHITE, BLUE & GREEN
Sara B, 26

SARA B: I was sort of older when I lost... well... I consider it older because people lose it fairly quickly nowadays. But I was in college, I was actually planning to wait until I was married. Yeah, that didn't happen.

SHAWN WICKENS: That's a pretty common plan though.

SB: Eventually like two months into my sophomore year after I had put this guy off for months I was like, "Oh, OK. OK. I'll be your girlfriend." He also hadn't had sex with anybody so it would have been both our first times and we were both sort of, "I don't know. Maybe we should." I talked about it with my roommate and she told me, "Oh. If you're going to, you have to go on the pill." I said, "Really? Is that what everybody does? OK." So without telling my boyfriend I went to the gynecologist and I had never been before. And I was like, "Uh, I need a prescription for birth control pills." I had to go to this class. It was creepy.

SW: Like a school gynecologist?

SB: Yeah, yeah. And it was really funny because we had to go to this class and there were all of these girls sitting in on this birth control pill seminar. So I went on the pill and I remember I told him. He came to my dorm room and I was like, "Look what I got." And he got really freaked out. He was like, "Well I don't even know if I want to have sex with you." And I was like, "Oh. OK." That was in October... I actually remember the actual date we had sex. It was November 28, and it was... 1998.
I'd been on the pill for like a month.

SW: You started taking them even though he freaked out?

SB: Yeah, yeah. So the whole story was... we hadn't planned on it, but I went to his off-campus apartment, he had made me dinner. Had some wine. His roommates were gone. He made me dinner. We had some wine and... we watched *Dances with Wolves* and started making out and we were all romantic so he was like, "I think we should make love," I think is what he called it. I was like, "OK." So we went to his room and... we were like just about there and he was like, "Oh, fuck. I don't have condoms so... Um. OK. Let's go into my roommate's room." We went to his roommate's room, went through his closet, literally tore apart his closet looking for condoms.

SW: Were you half-dressed at this point?

SB: I was completely undressed at this point, in his roommate's room. We finally found some and they were non-lubricated, which we were like, "Uh, OK. I guess that's fine." Went back to his room. And we did it, you know, missionary. I think he was like in and out maybe two or three times and then it was over. And I was like, "Oh. Was that? Oh... Cool." And he was like, "Let's have a cigarette."

SW: Were you even smokers?

(...and how not to)

SB: No. No his third roommate, the one we didn't take the condoms from, he was a smoker. We took his cigarettes and we were like, "Yeah, that's really sexy. Aren't you supposed to do something really sexy after you have sex?"

But then the funny thing was that the next day he made me a necklace because we had shared this really... special, you know...

SW: What was it made out of?

SB: It was beads. It was like... ohmigod. He was a very... all-American boy. So he made this red, white, and blue beaded necklace and then in the middle there was one green bead and that symbolized me because I really liked green. I might actually still have that. I don't know.

SW: Did you wear the necklace often or no?

SB: Ohmigod, every day. I was really cheesy about it too. I was like, "OK, I'm totally gonna marry you because we were both virgins and we lost our virginity together so." It actually lasted for a year. We still randomly communicate off and on.

> The next morning we had sex and she said the most flattering thing she could have possibly said and it has continued to give me confidence throughout the years. She looked at me and said, "Are you sure you've never had sex before?"
>
> *Russell, 20*
> *Land O' Lakes, Florida*

CONCEDING THE MATCH
Oliver, 31

I was very lucky to have a sweet, smart girl as a high school girlfriend because I didn't deserve her. I was a horny 17-year-old and I had verbally pressured her so much to go all the way that she came up with this system that, looking back on it was quite mature for two teenagers. We decided that the day she wanted to do it, while we were fooling around she would give me two taps on the back.

One afternoon we were hooking up in my bedroom and out of the blue she tapped me twice on the back. I said, "Really?" She didn't answer, she just tapped me again. That was that. We giggled a lot afterwards, which surprised us. I can remember telling her that maybe the first time isn't supposed to be too serious. It's supposed to be kind of fun and loose.

THE CALL OF THE WILD
Julie, 30

I was absolutely not considered in a sexual way by any male in high school. I begged six of the dorkiest guys to take me to prom and they all said, "No." So I was one of those girls who was accidentally forced to wait.

After high school I found out about this job up in Bethel, Alaska, rebuilding troughs that led up the side of waterfalls for salmon to swim up and get back to their breeding territory. My dad's dead and my mother's crazy so I had no trouble uprooting myself and traveling up north. I saved up money and I was as pure as a virgin snow when I arrived up there like Sam McGee from Tennessee*. I journeyed to Alaska intending to save the fish but I instead found out that more money was to be made in actually gutting and canning them, tending them from a boat off the Kuskokwim River.

On this fish boat of maybe three females and 86 males there was a baker named Mack. I was 19, he was 27 and Mack the Baker, in my 19-year-old sentimental mind, somewhat reminded me of Calvin from Calvin and Hobbes. Anyway I let it slip to Noreen the Cook who had lost like 90% of her arm in a cutlery accident, I accidentally let it slip to this untrustworthy cook Noreen that I thought Mack the Baker should be the man who devirginizes me. I thought it was time and I was in Alaska, the land of men. We were on a boat killing fish, it was a very primal setting. He was a Capricorn just like my dad.

Rumors spread and he caught wind of my yearning loins and cornered me one evening at the back end of the boat. He came up on me as I was gazing out at this beautiful sunset, like a backdrop from the movie musical *Oklahoma*. I was having a private, whimsical, weighted 19-year-old moment looking out at the sunset, all this beauty, and Mack the Baker cavalierly waltzes up and the first thing he ever said to me, which was the first thing he said to me in the six months I was there was, "So, I hear you want me to take your virginity." An enormous red blemish erupted on my cheeks as I tried to pretend that that utterance had not been uttered. It felt that at least 3,000 seconds had passed before he stated, "I don't think it's such a good idea."

Now I was a woman of integrity, even at 19. So I ignored the entire scenario. I had pretended none of it had ever happened. I conjured up in my mind that he was quite the asshole for coming up with this fantasy all on his own, even though I was the source of the saucy rumor to begin with.

Two weeks passed. I was working up in a box loft with Vera, an ex-prima ballerina from the Bolshoi Ballet. She said, "Mack is a dirty man. Mack is a dirty, dark, dirty man." I said to her, "I can't help it. He is the one to take my virginity and there's nothing that will stand in the way," except for time. And it took another whole two weeks before Mack the Baker showed up while I was on kitchen duty and blithely requested that I shave his head. I knew this was like my golden hour so I obliged. I shaved him like Curly from The Three Stooges, and then I got fucked in one of the sleeping niches in the boat quarters. It was great and I came. Somehow, somewhere that 19-year-old girl knew that he was the man to do it and it may have been the best sex I have ever had and I never spoke to him again.

*from the poem "The Cremation of Sam McGee" by Robert Service

(...and how not to)

THE ACCIDENTAL TOURIST
Gary, 45

My dad and I were traveling in Europe with his mother. We had planned to get her through at least Germany and my dad figured it was only $120 more to go to his hometown with his mother, so we continued on to Beirut. I ended up going to school there because I had stayed past the time when my school started back in Texas.

I'm 15 and they started me in the seventh grade and then they backed me up to the third grade, then they backed me up to first grade, then they said, "You need to learn the alphabet," so they put me in kindergarten.

I'm 15 in a Beirut kindergarten and then I met Ahisma. She lived around the corner, two blocks from us and we would ride the bus together. We rode the bus together every day. After we had ridden together for about six months she began tutoring me in Arabic. I would go to her place after school and study with her and after a few lessons we had our first kiss. She decided that she liked me enough that we became better neighbors. And one thing led to another and... let me tell you... I miss her. She's dead now; she got killed by a car bomb back in 1978. Yeah, it's just one of those horrible things.

But she was my tutor, it had nothing to do with school. It had to do with the fact that we were neighbors, and we just got along. She was three years older than I was and I was proud because I was dating an 18-year-old. My grandmother would look at me and say, "Where are you going?" "I'm going to my teacher's house." "Oh, OK." Grandma thought everything was innocent and cool. Yeah right, I was really studying anatomy by Braille. It was just a natural passage.

She was a great teacher. Let me tell you, she was a great teacher. She taught me some things I ain't forgotten yet. And let me tell you, I ain't had no complaints.

We kept in touch until the day that she got killed. And unfortunately, like I said... the son of a bitches turned a parked car into a bomb. She was walking by, heading for the bus stop and the damn thing went off and she's gone. But she'll always be in my heart. I couldn't go for the funeral but I got to go in 1980 and '81 with the National Guard, I was a translator. And 249 of my friends are gone because of the time we spent over there. But you know, I'm here. And I have the memories and... Ahisma, I miss you.

In high school a friend of ours set it up for me to watch one of his wrestling tournaments... and I watched him and there was just like a connection – instant connection. Don't know what it was. If I believe in destiny, or soul mates... I'd say it's there.
Angela, 37
Dayton, Oregon

THE SOUVENIR
Cindy, 48

The first time I saw him I was probably 12. I've always had a fascination with cars because I grew up in a car family. My uncles raced cars, my brothers raced cars so I had a thing for fast cars; I'm still that way. I would see this guy driving up and down the street in his yellow Camaro. That's how I met him, by seeing him in that car.

When I was 15 I was with my girlfriends and he drove by my house on his way to pick up his fiancé. He made a u-turn, came back and picked us up and he bought beer for us. After that he started just coming over, calling on me, taking me out and we started dating.

Here I am a 15-year-old girl dating a 20-year-old man. He had a really good job so while my girlfriends were lucky if they were even taken to a McDonald's, he was taking me out to really nice restaurants every Friday night. We were going out to movies, dancing, I mean I was madly in love.

My father was deceased at the time so I just had my mom. She knew I was seeing an older guy and she was not pleased to say the least. My mother grew up in a different era, she was 42 when she had me, I had brothers who were 20 years older than me. Nowadays that's kind of like the norm having children later in life, but back then it was rare. So she was not happy about it but unsure how to deal with it.

But I was crazy in love with this guy because he had a canary yellow 1970 Camaro... and he was hot. He kept telling me, "I'm gonna get you. I'm gonna get you. I'm gonna get you." I was like, "No. I can't do this. I can't do this. I can't do this." But you're a 15-year-old girl, you still have those feelings and you want to do it. At the same time I had my mother telling me what I should do, what I shouldn't do, who I needed to be. I was trying to be a good person but after five months of this conflict, we were at the drive-in one night and... we did it.

I can't remember the movie that was playing, but I do know we were at the Skyway Drive-In near Warren, Ohio. We did it in the backseat of his car there was some blood. He had this t-shirt on so he took off his shirt and cleaned up the business with it. This is pretty creepy and gross but I still have the shirt. My present husband doesn't know this but it's in my underwear drawer.

Anyway we had sex three times that night and I had heard from girlfriends that it's terrible the first time. I didn't feel that way at all. It was unbelievable. We had sex three times, it was just amazing to me.

What ended up happening though, because I was so much younger than him, I couldn't go to bars because the legal age in Ohio was 18. I couldn't go to bars so I couldn't compete, but he could go out and meet lots of girls. It got so I couldn't handle that anymore, even though he wanted to continue dating, so we broke up. I actually ended up marrying somebody else. That didn't work out, it broke up so I did end up getting back together with him, the first boyfriend and we did get married. Then, unfortunately, after nine years of marriage for whatever reason we couldn't make it last.

But looking back, it was very enthralling, very exciting and I'll never forget that. I'll end up forgetting a lot of things but I'll never forget that. It was a life-changing event and I still remember it like it was last night. I still think about being in the back seat of his Camaro, the one I first saw him driving, at the Skyway Drive-In each time I pull his shirt out of my underwear drawer.

(...and how not to)

THE NERD AND THE BULLY
Devin, 34

I'm from Dayton, Oregon, which is a small town, little farming town outside Portland. I was kind of a geeky kid in high school – a little guy. Didn't get a lot of attention from girls, but that's OK. Then I started dating a girl when I was a sophomore in high school who was a little bit more wild than I was.

We went to school together, obviously, and the first time I met her was in fifth grade and even though right now she's five feet tall, she was five feet tall back then too. She was the big kid in school, and the bully. She became the cute little thing later. We started dating in high school and I guess I was a little surprised by how sexually aggressive she was. Not that she had a lot of experience either but I guess she knew what she liked and luckily it happened to be me.

I think it was, well OK, I know it was June 14th, 1986. Almost 20 years ago. Four months and 16 days after we started dating. We were in the basement of my parents' house, with my parents home of course. And yeah, it lasted for maybe a minute. The build-up lasted for about two hours, but the whole thing lasted for about a minute. And she was understanding of that because then it happened again another 15 minutes later and it lasted a little longer that time.

I guess it was a weird situation. It was, you know... it was scary. I know women talk about losing their virginity as a big deal but I guess for me it was a big deal as well.

We didn't have plans to do it. I knew we were working towards that. In fact she offered that up to me a couple weeks before and I had, embarrassed to say now, turned it down because I was scared. But I have to be honest, it changed my life. It changed the way everybody thought about me at school, how I saw myself. Everything.

I really knew that I liked her a lot. I knew we had a definite connection but I didn't know we'd eventually get married. All through high school and college, I got lots of pressure from my friends to be with somebody else but I guess I just knew. I knew she was the one. I guess I got lucky that the first one was *the one*. Some people might say I got unlucky because I haven't been able to sleep with a bunch of women, but I know I don't need to.

We got married when I was 21. We've got two kids now, one is 7, one is 2. But as far as when I have to talk to them about sex... I don't really believe in waiting for marriage. I think being married to someone who you are sexually incompatible with would be a huge mistake. So, you know, they need to know something about that. I guess that makes me a liberal father. I'm not sure. I think one thing I'll always want to tell both my son and my daughter is that sex is a serious thing and because it is so serious you should make sure it works before you make that commitment.

But looking back... my first time was exciting and quick and scary. And everything I'd heard that it was emotionally, for girls, that's the way it was for me.

I SLIPPED INSIDE HER
Ben, 19

I'm from Mankato. It's a rural town in south central Minnesota. I started dating this girl when I was 15 years old and we were together for like a year and a half total. For the last nine months of it, she moved an hour and a half away to go to college in the Twin Cities.

It was actually kind of interesting because it was a slow development over months and months and months. Every other weekend or so she would either come down and visit me or I would go up to visit her. The very first weekend after she started school was the very first time I touched her breasts. Then like two weekends later it was the first time one of us took our shirts off. Two weeks after that we took a shower together in the common bathroom of her dorm. No one was awake so it was a slow time for showering when we wouldn't be bothered. We were naked but we didn't have sex. That's very hard to do after you've lost your virginity but before – it's a lot easier. Plus we were accustomed to the slow build of things.

Finally one weekend she came down to visit me at home. I had a fireplace in our basement and luckily it was kind of cold that night so we built a fire. One of our big things was giving massages to each other and she had surprised me with massage oils. There was massaging going on for probably an hour and a half or two hours. Then it was kind of funny how easily it happened.

Usually when you see things in the movies "just happening" or there's a talk about how it's all some weird moral dilemma you're like, "Oh that's total bullshit." But it actually did turn out to be the idyllic sort of thing. One minute she was on her stomach without any clothes on and I was massaging her, and then the next moment she rolled over and looked into my eyes and... no words, it was just kind of understood. We had sex on my basement floor.

Before I even started dating her, one of my friends had told me that even if you're not going to use it, you should always have a condom on you in case anyone else should need it. Like if you're at a party or anything it's good to have protection on hand for somebody. That had become my policy for a really long time so I had a condom.

It was really good. We were just two really curious, oiled up, yet strangely responsible teenagers.

(...and how not to)

MY BUDDY LIST
Dennis, 27

When I was 19, I met another man in an AOL chat room about game shows because as long as I've been alive I've been absolutely obsessed with game shows – things like *The Price is Right* and the old *Match Game* and whatever else. Well this man flew in from Austin, Texas, to Maryland where we spent the weekend at a Red Roof Inn and he gave me a blowjob and that's all.

So that was the first guy who sucked on my dick. Losing your virginity is a lot like losing your innocence. So that episode was losing my innocence. That was me breaking into the gay scene and becoming myself. But to be perfectly honest, I lost my full virginity at 26 with my husband. That was the first time that I really got fucked.

I met my husband at this very bar. I had met him on my birthday and like three months after that we decided that we were going to buy a house together. All of my friends and family were very much opposed to it because they had never met him and they thought I was making a rash decision. I was making a rash decision absolutely but I was thinking with my heart and so I went with it. I have no regrets. None. And it's all worked out very well.

First came the anal sex, then the house. But yeah, when I met him I had never been fucked or fucked. Never had sex with a woman, never had any interest in having sex with a woman.

He is actually three years younger than me and he's had a lot of experiences. He studied acting in New York and he slept with everyone under the sun. I thought I was a whore until I met him. Luckily neither of us were unfortunate enough to contract any diseases. But he was very much more experienced than me and he totally eased me into it. He eased me into anal sex with one finger at a time and he even made me a mix CD with songs pertinent to us back then and he titled it "One Finger at a Time." I had never had anyone else put his dick inside me and I've never put my dick inside of anyone else and I have to say that I am very, very, very happy and not looking to stray.

Having someone who knew what to do certainly helped with the physical aspect of it. He was very understanding and very patient. I can't emphasize that enough – very patient. Because... when you put things in your butt... it hurts. Eventually you grow to get used to that sort of thing but it takes lots of work.

He was living at a repertory theatre and that was the first time I had sex was in his bed that he was renting backstage and it was amazing. The fireworks were there.

THE VELVET REVOLUTION
Lienhart, 38

I'm from the Czech Republic and this happened back in 1989. At that time there was this huge change that began to happen that resulted in the ultimate removal of the Communist Party as the only source of power, the holder of power. The whole event started as a wave of public disagreement that was sparked by the university students.

I was a senior studying biology at Purkyne University in Brno which is a central city in Moravia in the eastern part of the Czech Republic, or what used to be the central part of Czechoslovakia. I was about to finish my undergraduate degree when all of the students went on strike, occupational strike. Suddenly we went from simply studying at this institution of learning to being in charge and we were doing political activism. It was an exciting time to be there. And it just so happened that one of my closest friends had brought his girlfriend into our midst and she became a member of our core group, about a dozen people or so and myself who helped to organize protests and marches and walkouts. She and I had kind of struck this relationship, an interest in each other. We had this sudden outpouring of emotion and closeness and you have to realize that to go out and put your entire life and prospects on the line for the future – it was a pretty heavy deal. And to find somebody who's going to just sort of carry you through that to the next state for our country, or even the next morning was an incredible thing in its own right. This girl, Věra was the one I have given my virginity.

Really it was just a fling for her although I had wished and wanted it to be more than that. I still think back on losing my virginity in what essentially had been a lecture hall for organic chemistry. It was during the occupational strike at a time when me and my friends were helping to decide the future of our country. No matter how cynical you might be looking at that era or even the current state of the world, looking back at that specific moment, it was a grand thing.

The truth is, is that she and my friend got together later again. And later still she left him and went back to a man who had been her high school sweetheart and the last thing I knew before I left the country and moved to America was that she got married to that man and had a child. I last saw my friend the summer before last. He's gone on with his life; we're still good friends.

To put it in his words, and I will never really be certain whether he knew what really happened at that time with me and Věra, but later on when we were reminiscing, he said very simply and succinctly, "The revolution taught Europe how to handle women." And that may not have really been the whole truth but it certainly took away some of our naïveté, individually and as a society. I don't think it made me less of a romantic but I think it made me, at the cost of some pain, a wiser man. And if that's not an achievement then nothing is.

(...and how not to)

POETRY IN MOTION
Julius, 41

When did I lose my virginity? It happened so fast. Mmm... trying to think back through my sex life. It started I guess... before my puberty. So then... yeah, the official one would have been this lovely girl. Her father was the headmaster at the local school. We were both in the same school... and... oh, it was wonderful. We took the whole day off... you know, little kiddie stories. We just were off playing in the fields of Ireland. Got off school for the summer and spent the whole summer making love. But school didn't end, I guess. She taught me how to make love.

We... we... we gaffed off school... got in her car, and then got out of the city and into the country... and I was shaking like an idiot. She was like the leader... beautiful, voluptuous girl. And... I couldn't get out of her breasts. She went down on me... it was all over. It was very embarrassing. And then... after another while... awkwardly I mounted her... and I... slipped into her. It was warm... gorgeous... ah, it's coming all back now. And it was over like that, *snap*.

I'm thinking... trying to get into the mood of that time... it was all very slutty... there was no love involved at all. Just pure lust, testosterone and hormones and... I woke up in a puddle of confusion. I saw her naked body... and the head of my penis was ripped to pieces. And the faces that people make when they make love... it's like a donkey - the most ugly faces in the world.

We were done and we drove out of the country, into the city. I think we had a bite to eat and had a swim. And then... we couldn't keep our hands off each other for the whole summer. It wasn't like, "Hey you wanna go out somewhere and do something?" it was, "Let's go and fuck. Let's go and fuck." We were fucking on top of wardrobes, in supermarkets, everywhere... experimenting all over the place. And the more risqué the better.

And of course we thought it was forever. But... she basically fucked my brains out for the summer. Then she moved on, and I... masturbated for the winter.

She was going to be a concert pianist, and I was going to be a world famous artist. Then she became a music teacher and I became an underground, dropout artist in the Chelsea Hotel. *Heh*... what a time.

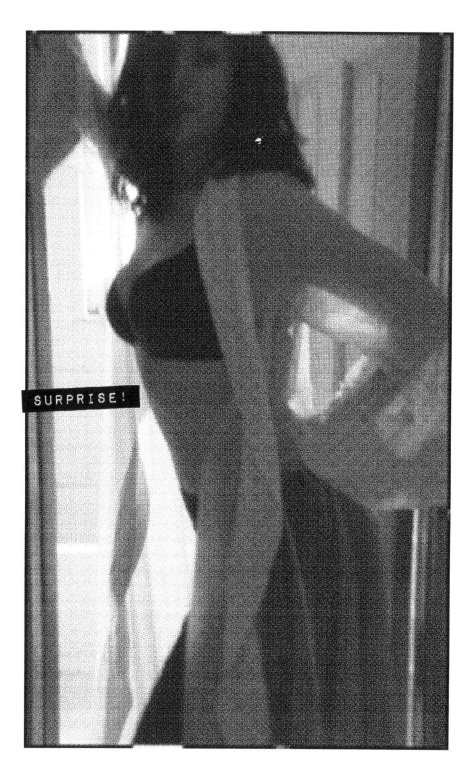

(...and how not to)

"JUST FELL INTO IT"

7

It's a common feeling to get swept up in the moment during the first time, even more so when your mind is racing, "I can't believe this is happening." Some people plan for the moment and stress to make everything perfect. Others just luck into it. Some first times are engineered, others are serendipitous.

    A few more same sex-stories appear in this chapter as opposed to other chapters. When you grow up heterosexual and you're dating, even if you're just around members of the opposite sex, the possibility of sex, no matter how slight, is right in front of you. But when your sexuality is a secret, the opportunities are hidden and make for more spontaneous or accidental experiences.

REMEMBER THAT FRIEND OF YOURS?
Craig, 25

I was a late bloomer. It was my second year at Penn State when I finally became very dissatisfied with how college was going for me at that point. I was involved with a few girls but never got up the mustard, the "minimals," as they say, to finally carry it out.

We had a party at my apartment and a bunch of friends were there. My younger brother went to Penn State too and he brought along one of his friends, Janet. They were in the same year. Everyone is hanging out. It's the various college ways and means of partying, especially at Penn State. Various drugs and stuff involved. Mostly alcohol and pot but very large quantities of the two.

After the party started to wind down I went to the living room and started watching *American Beauty*. I was changing from mathematics to a film studies major so this serious movie was just one of those movies in college I was inspired by. Janet, my brother's friend, wanted to watch the movie with me so it was just the two of us.

It's the end of the night, as I said, and time is winding down. All of my roommates are passed out in their rooms. She's sitting there on the couch next to me and I figured something was going to happen. Her head went down in my lap and there was nothing holding us back at that point. I mean, it was obvious. It's three in the morning and the room was pitch black except for the television. I guess she was just looking for affection. From what my brother later told me she wasn't much enjoying her experience at college. She wasn't finding her place and I think she was just looking for someone who seemed confident with their surroundings.

She came close and cuddled. I thought, "Let's just do this, get it out of the way." So we started kissing.

I don't believe it was her first time. I think for her it was just a college hook-up. Maybe she was under the impression I was a seasoned veteran and I didn't tell her anything that would make her think any different. We started going at it on the couch and it was a terrible couch. A college piece-of-trash couch. No sort of comfort involved whatsoever. It was hard to move around. Finally I sat back and let her get on top of me and because of the alcohol and drugs I was having trouble physically responding.

We're going at it and finally I'm building up, I'm building up and I say to her, "Oh, I'm about to cum." She's out of it as well and since we were going for so long and we were so messed up, she must've heard, "I can't." She gets up and starts apologizing, "Oh, I'm sorry. I'm sorry." I was sitting there dumbfounded by the situation. I was thinking, "No. Don't. Stop," but at that point it was already ruined. So I just separated from her, let her sleep on the couch and I took the floor.

The next morning everyone woke up and just saw us on separate places, you know, my roommate was hooking up with his girl in our bedroom and she felt bad that I got relocated and got stuck sleeping on the floor. Little did she know that I was having sex with her friend in the living room.

I'd see the girl I slept with on the street here and there, waking around campus and such. My brother, Chris, would talk to me about, "Yeah, I saw her the other day." And I'd be like, "How did that go?" I've still never had the brass to tell him I had sex with his good friend.

(...and how not to)

THE ACCIDENTAL JOHN
Marcus, 33

There was this girl who lived in my neighborhood in Makersfield, Northern England, and for a pound she would take you to her room and let you look at her with her clothes off. I was 13. She was 15 or 16.

I lied to my dad and told him I needed to get a book for school so he gave me a fiver. And everyone in the neighborhood was going over this girl's family's house. The parents were out, her younger brother was downstairs and she was upstairs in the bedroom.

So it was an investment really. And it was worth it, haven't done anything like that again. Everyone else was just looking, but the five-pound note got a little bit more. She saw that and it was full-on sex. Kept my Doc Martens on and that was that. Everybody else kind of knew something was going on 'cause I was in there a little longer than everyone else.

My dad asked me about the book as I was supposed to give him the receipt, which I told him I lost as was par for the course.

I CALL SHOTGUN
Curtis, 49

It was with an acquaintance, a friend of my nephew's. She and I weren't boyfriend and girlfriend, she was just someone I knew. We had gone out to a concert one night. We were young and we were out partying.

My nephew and I are very close in age. He's actually six months older than I am. My older sister was pregnant and then I came along – an accident.

So we're out drinking and we're in my nephew's Trans Am, which was an easy car to pick up girls in. We went to a lot of concerts back in the day. My first concert was, I think, Vinegar Joe with Mahogany Rush, but I don't think this happened after that show. We had a long drive at the end of the night all the way back Mobile, Alabama. We had a good time and then we partied and drank the whole ride back to Lucedale, Mississippi. We were riding around drinking just like always and we just decided to stop at a creek bank. I could sense what was going on, it was obvious but I was scared about it.

I don't remember whose idea it was, maybe it was a mutual decision but somebody said, "Hey, let's go skinny dipping." Soon enough we were butt naked on a creek side in Mississippi basically half in and half out of the water, like an amphibian experience. Not quite as romantic as *From Here to Eternity*.

Who slept with who was as much determined by who you were sitting next to in the car as much as anything else. It was very indiscriminate. She was a fairly aggressive young lady and we came together more as an act of nature than anything else.

It was wild the way it happened. And it was my first time and I was anxious and it was kind of anti-climactic, but sort of not. It was more just weird for how detached it was. Had we not been partying and drinking it probably never would have happened.

AWAKENING
Damon, 26

When I was 18 or 19 I was in the military at Fort Knox, Kentucky. One of the other recruits came over to my bunk and called me by my last name, "Wake up. I gotta talk to you." It was about three o'clock in the morning and we only got maybe four hours of sleep anyway, so I was like, "Yo, take your ass to bed." He said, "OK," only I didn't hear him walk away. He didn't move. I turned over and he's like, "All right." I'm like, "All right, what?" And he goes, "All right I'll suck your dick."

I was on the top bunk. I pulled my dick out and he started working it. I changed my mind and tried to pull away but he didn't let me. He sucked my dick and it was the best suck I ever had. There were 50 people in our bay and they had to have known what was going on, but it was weird, nobody said anything.

I was the greatest, straightest man before that happened. I had nothing to do with homosexuals, so when it happened it was, I don't know, dynamic... different. After that I was hooked.

MERRY XXXMAS
Randi, 23

I was 16 and a half and it was the day after Christmas. I was with my best friend Bella and we decided to go next door to Heather's apartment, who I've known since I was two. It was me, my best friend Bella, Heather, and her boyfriend Daniel. We were totally alone drinking vodka. It was the first time I had ever consumed alcohol.

I can't remember what game we were playing, one of those games you act out stuff like "truth or dare", but Heather said something like, "Hey, how about we have a threesome," and I was like, "OK." And it quickly turned into a threesome with me, Daniel, and Heather. Bella sat in the back corner and watched. It was very surreal.

We took off our clothes, and I fingered Heather for a bit. We all fooled around for probably about an hour and a half with Bella just watching the whole time. Then it was mainly Bella and Heather watching me have sex with Heather's boyfriend. But it seemed everyone was having a good time.

The next day Bella asked if I felt different. I was like, "Not really. I just feel like I got something out of the way." But it was very awkward for me because I had known Heather for so long. Still every time I see her it's in the back of my mind, "Wow, OK. I had sex with your boyfriend while you watched." Very weird.

I ran into the boyfriend two years after it happened. He put his arm around me and was like, "Hey, Randi. How you doing?" I was just like, "I'm great. Go away."

(...and how not to)

THERESE'S BIG ADVENTURE
Therese, 36

It was my sophomore year, so that would've been '84. I had just turned 15 and my friend Kimberly and I went to go see *Pee-Wee's Big Adventure*. I was a huge Pee-Wee fan so I had to go see this movie. So we went and we loved it... well I loved it. We came back to my house around 10 o'clock, 11 o'clock at night and got a call that a bunch of our friends were at a party up the street.

Kimberly and I walked the quarter of a mile, half mile down to this kid's house for the party. We get there and everyone was like really, really drunk. As soon as we arrived my friend Job pulled me aside and started explaining to me that out of all our group of friends there were only two virgins left – me and Heath, who had been my best friend in grade school. Heath and I were the only two left so Job was like, "Look. Therese. It's kind of retarded at this point. You should probably just do it." Before then I had never really felt embarrassed by the fact that I had waited.

Here's the back-story on why I was the last girl in my group of friends to lose her virginity... or why they did it first. We had this other friend who was an only child, really, really brilliant – she's like a Ph.D. in biology now. Growing up she was really wild and really, really slutty.

The previous summer she picked up some dude at this resort hotel near where we lived. It used to be like an old Playboy club so they had a pool and everything and it was real swanky. Her dad used to take her there to go swimming. As I heard it, she was walking around the arcade one day and this dude, like this townie kid, threw her just a little bit of attention... she wasn't particularly pretty... he threw her just a little bit of attention and he took her into the stairwell and fucked the hell out of her.

Subsequently she fucked all his friends, I'm talking within the first month that they knew each other. Then the friends of his that she didn't fuck, she pimped out all of our other friends to fuck the guy's other friends.

They would have these massive hotel parties, the same hotel. I got asked but I refused to go. I found the whole thing very distasteful. My friend Kimberly the one who I saw *Pee-Wee's Big Adventure* with... yeah, she lost her virginity to some dude like five years older than us who drove a car. Not for me.

Well, that's why I was the last one left and for whatever reason Heath was left too. And I guess everyone else was feeling really braggy, you know like, "Ohh, we've done it... like a million times." For all I know, this proposal could have been Heath's idea all along and he asked Job to bring it up to me.

So Heath and I spoke and he was all, "You want to?" I was like, "I guess. You want to?" And he was like, "I guess." At that point I didn't have a crush on him, but back in fifth grade I did. But he was a cute guy and we had been friends for forever.

Someone gave Heath a condom and sent us off to the privacy of the basement rec room of this split-level house. That was the first time he and I made out or anything. Afterward, Kimberly came down to the basement and I remember her asking me all comforting-like, "Aww, are you O.K.?" I went, "Yeah, I guess." I know it's cliché but I remember thinking, "Was that it?"

It was awful and I don't have a daughter but if I ever do I would hope that she'd have a very experienced person for her first because my guy didn't know what he was doing and it was awful. It was just so... perfunctory... would be the best word to describe it. I mean I only did it with Heath because this other guy Job brought it up.

I was expecting it to be painful and it was. It was painful over and over and over again. I guess some girls bleed more than others, I wasn't all that particularly bleedy.

When we came out it was kind of like a celebration at the town square like, "It's official!" You know there was some backslapping and some high fiving. There was like a chorus of, "Hey! All right!" from all our friends. Then that was it. I was a bit disappointed.

The weird thing was afterwards, we did it a few more times. It wasn't any better. I'm not sure what Heath was thinking but I overheard him talking to a mutual friend and I heard Heath use the term "a piece of trim," and I was the piece of trim he was referring to. And I thought, "Are you kidding me? He called me his 'piece of trim'?" I wasn't really offended so much as surprised. I had never been called a piece of trim before. I've never even been called that since. It sounded like something you learn from reading Playboy and he was so not that guy, but whatever.

But that's it. It was so clumsy and neither of us knew what to do. It was weird but I'm glad it was with him because... I mean he was at my first wedding and everything. We stayed friends so he was a nice guy in the end.

> I said flat out, "I think you should show me your penis." It was bold because I was so young. He said, "There's about a zero percent chance of that happening." We've since talked about how funny it was that it went from a zero percent chance to eventually going all the way.
>
> *Kathryn, 24*
> *Crystal Lake, Illinois*

A GIFT FOR BOTH OF US
Anthony, 21

I was 16 years old and my first girlfriend, my first everything and I were going out for four or five months. My girlfriend was the virgin of the group and she said she wouldn't have intercourse until she got married. It was coming up on Valentine's Day and she wanted me to get a tongue ring.

The first time I used the tongue ring on her, she wanted the sex right away. I didn't even have to talk her into it. She was on top of me, I was working her orally and the tongue ring pushed it over the edge. For a second there was no condom, and then we got one. It's almost like I tripped and fell into my first time.

After then we talked about, "Should we have sex again?" We had already had sex for the first time, she was ready now and we basically had a lot of sex after that.

A couple of my friends joked about getting a tongue ring because I was the first of any of them to have sex. Getting that tongue ring was the right decision.

(...and how not to)

KNOCK, KNOCK. WHO'S THERE?
George, 22

It was totally a one night stand, like hard-core. This guy Johnny who was friends with my older sister would always come over to our house and bring over girls he met from the bar. My sister didn't even live at the house anymore but he still used our house as a crash pad. So he brings this lady over but she's totally not interested in him at all. I was sleeping on the couch and woke me up when they came over. And she was just all about me. She laid down next to me on the couch and he left. We made out for a second and then she started, you know, she went down my pants, got on and whatnot. It's funny, I've told this story a million times but I can't explain why it happened. It lasted maybe five seconds. She was 34. I was 14. About a 20-year difference.

Johnny totally hooked me up, inadvertently. I let them in and she was hot but he could see that she wanted me so he gave it the go ahead. You know, he wasn't a virgin - he was like a 30-year-old man. If he was 16 he wouldn't have been as generous.

She actually told me it was the best sex she ever had. I didn't really believe it. I mean, I still don't. A young guy like that? Maybe she was letting me down gently or maybe she was endowing me with confidence.

I wish I could say it was special and everything. It happened so fast I didn't really have time to enjoy it. Pretty much right when she opened the door it was obvious that because of how young I was that she wanted to do me. If I had been an older guy, I don't think it would have happened. She just wanted to rob the cradle - that's my take on it.

FEMALE EXPLORATION
Natasha, 34

A couple of years ago I lost my virginity to a woman. And she is the only woman I've ever had in my life. Her name was Andi.

I was vacationing in Miami and I had just got divorced. One of my best friends was trying to hook me up with guys and I was not really into it. We decided to sail from Miami to the Bahamas. We were a group of 10 people on a beautiful boat. He later told me that he paid this woman a couple of thousand dollars to do me, but I didn't know that. She ended up falling in love with me.

We were all on the boat and we were doing ecstasy and coke and weed and champagne and the yacht was beautiful, the ocean, everything and the next thing I know I have this really beautiful, sexy Pocahontas-looking woman, Andi, going after me. She was my first woman experience and it lasted three days and it was fantastic. I have never had a girl since then and I don't think ever will. I'm not really into girls, I'm really hetero. But I have to say that that experience was fantastic. It was the first time I had a dildo used on me. It was different because I'm not one to masturbate. I'm very active, I'm too busy with my work and music to do stuff like that. But that experience was great as well... both experiences, the first man and the first woman were both fantastic.

SURPRISE
Jason, 40

I was the guy in school, when asked, "Do you masturbate?" didn't raise his hand. I didn't even know it was an option. I wasn't as frustrated as I would be years later, after I realized what I had been missing.

I lost my virginity at 19. It's about the right age to lose your virginity, I guess. We were having a party at Ted's house. I was going to community college and we invited a lot of women over.

This party was going along and then late in the night, Ted and this woman disappeared into one of the back bedrooms. Someone was looking for him so I went around knocking on the back bedroom doors. I walked into this one room, my friend wasn't around but there she was this strange woman in a teddy. Ted and I looked very similar to each other. She looked at me and said, "Fuck me." So I did.

It was on Ted's sister's bed and the sheets were very, very, very soiled. So he had to explain to his sister what happened in there. My buddy was also upset because I had locked the door and I think at one point he was trying to get back in.

She was so drunk she didn't care who it was. I mean, she came to a party wearing a teddy underneath her clothes. But I did do the right thing and gave her a ride home. But yeah, it was with a stranger I walked in on at a party. Didn't even know her name. I think it's one of the reasons I've turned out to be less of a romantic.

THIS ONE TIME, AT JOB CORPS...
Ruby, 24

I'm bisexual. And I've always known that I'm bisexual. And I really don't have a preference between girls and boys. I love them both. So I lost my virginity to a boy at Job Corps on Valentine's Day. I lost my virginity to a girl that same year in Job Corps.

I didn't know it was going to happen. I was supposed to go home for the weekend with a different friend but she never showed up. And this other friend of mine from Job Corps was leaving. I was like, "What the hell. I've got the weekend pass. I'll go too." I had sex with the woman who came to pick up that other friend. I left with them and I started giving her a massage while she was driving the car. She had somebody switch and they drove, and she sat in the backseat with me and we just started making out and it just got heavier and heavier.

Eventually when we got to her house we went all the way. Her husband watched so that was pretty neat. She said I did a really good job. They were nudists anyway so we just stripped down and stayed naked for most of the weekend.

(see page 116)

(...and how not to)

INCOGNITO
Clay, 44

I was invited to a Halloween party by a friend. It was a gay Halloween party and I didn't really know anyone there. I was 22 and not out of the closet yet. I came from a strict family and my mother told us kids that if we had sex before we got married, our arms would fall off. Very old school. It was years before I could come out to my siblings. Because of my background, I held on to my virginity for quite awhile.

The whole party was basically naked. I was dressed as a Banshee, one of those Irish folk monsters that screams all the time. I was wearing basically a loincloth, my eyes were blacked out and I had hair glued all over my body. I looked really scary, but I was basically naked too. I got real drunk on these shots called Jellybeans, which were seven different liquors all layered together. I blacked out and the next thing I remember was coming to in the middle of a ménage a trois, and I had somebody at both ends. I wouldn't assume I was forced into it because I was having a good time. Two boyfriends decided to get me involved in something. They coaxed me into a bedroom and I was so drunk I didn't know what was going on until I came to. The one guy's costume was just a towel and shaving cream on his face. I can't recall what the other guy was wearing. It was mayhem. It was great. I was having fun and then I blacked out again.

The next morning I was shaved head to toe. It went from being a threesome to a gag. I had absolutely no hair left on my body. I guess they wanted to see how much of my hair was real and how much was glued on. It was a sleazy way to lose it but I thought it was funny. I saw the guys again a few times but they were in a committed relationship. I was just a fling for the night.

> She grabbed my hand and took me to the other side of the basketball court, to the women's locker room. She said, "I hear you're a virgin. Virgins aren't allowed to start on the defensive squad." Then we fucked in the women's locker room.
>
> *Tim, 28*
> *Piedmont, Oklahoma*

ON THE DOWN LOW
James, 44

My sister and I went to the same high school. She was two years ahead of me and we both went on to the University of Pittsburgh. I'd say about 78% of her graduating class went to the University of Pittsburgh and about 50% of my graduating class went there as well. Her boyfriend from high school also went there, so they had been there for two years prior to me.

I had always felt some strange sort of, not so much sexual attraction, but I would always catch long stares from my sister's boyfriend. I would turn and he would be in on me, just staring.

When I got to college I lived in a co-ed dorm – every other floor was boy, girl, boy, girl. They housed everyone in chronological order. Our last name started with a "D" and so did my sister's boyfriend's. So my room was on the same floor as Simon's room.

Once in awhile I'd hang out in his dorm room and at one point there was a real nice girl, Sherry, in his room who I thought he had something going on with. The three of us were drinking and stuff and Simon got out this book called, *Total Massage*. We're flipping through it, we ate some mushrooms you know, we're feeling all cozy, "Let's try these massages." So everybody's clothes came off and we're all trying these massages on each other, these sexual massages.

So it was my sister's boyfriend, the girl, and myself. Nothing really sexually happened for the three of us, but before we knew it, it was like 7 o'clock in the morning. She jumped up, "I have class," and ran out of the room. I close the door behind her and all we have on is our underwear and I turn around and Simon is raging a full-on hard-on, like a baby's arm. This guy played football for the Pitt Panthers. He was a quarterback, like a buck eighty-five, 6'8" – beautiful, a body made of granite. It startled me. I was trying to ignore it but he was very, very definite about what he was feeling. My skinny, track-runner legs were shaking in my shoes. I was like, "What?" And he's dead staring at me. He tells me, "I want to fuck you." And I'm like, "Well that's not going to happen. Hey, I don't do that. You're scaring me."

Meanwhile, you know, I was really turned on for the first time in my life, like really turned on. There was this naked man, a male's body, looking at me with raging hormones and beautiful muscle tone. There's this Adonis in front of me and I'm thinking, "Well here's my chance to actually have sex with another man." Completely negating the fact that he's my sister's boyfriend. I think to myself, "Who the hell will know?" I said, "OK. We can have sex but you're not fucking me with that... that, that thing. That weapon."

He picked me up with one arm, muscles all over the place and he throws me on the mattress. He jumps on top of me, he's grinding his body and he blows his whole load all over me. Meanwhile I was just getting started. "Oh that was good," he moans. And I'm like, "That was it?" He was like, "What?" as he's wiping the cum off his dick. I said, "Is that it?! If that's it I don't want to be gay!" and I ran out of his room.

(...and how not to)

    The next day I walked out of my dorm and it felt like the whole entire world knew what happened. I saw my sister and she had this look on her face, this, "I know what you did last night" look. I was like, "Bonnie, are you, uh… ready to go to class?" She was like very kind of persnickety, "Are you? Ready to go?" I was like, "What's the matter?" "Oh, nothing. How did you sleep?" I'm like, "Oh, shit. She knows," like an intuitive thing.

    I ran into the guy out at the bars a few years after we graduated. It was different. I was more mature and I understood better who I was. "What are you doing tonight?" I asked him. "I want to fuck you," he whispered in my ear. We went to his place and at that point it was five years after our first encounter. We had some really hot, hot, hot sex. I mean like deep, hot sex. He fucked me. He really fucked me. And I'm not one for getting fucked, it was just because we had that history and it was the mental turn-on that worked me up to the point to let him. It was really hot and I knew after that one time it would never happen again. He was just fucking me like he just had to do it, and he did it.

    I never spoke a word about any of me and Simon with my sister. She had once mentioned to me, "You know what? I think Simon was gay all those years." I just said, "Oh, yeah? Wow. What makes you think that? I wasn't hanging out with him… that much." And I left it at that.

> After we realized that we had done it… it was almost like she dropped a quarter. She dealt with it like it was change that dropped out of her pocket. Made me feel like an asshole and OK with it at the same time.
>
> *Vincent, 25*
> *Burlington, Vermont*

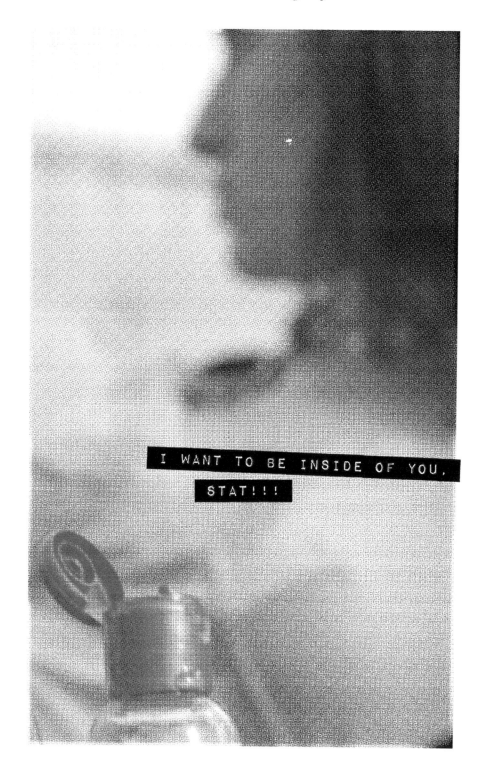

(...and how not to)

"I HAVE TWO RUBBERS; WEAR THEM BOTH, IT WILL DESENSITIZE YOU."

8

At the end of *American Pie* when Jason Biggs' character, Jim, is on the verge of making good on his pact to lose his virginity by prom night, his date tells him to wear two condoms because she is aware of his history of finishing early – an embarrassing fact of which most of his classmates are aware.

In spite of the less than ideal lead-in, Jim seems to perform without much trouble. And even if it's awkward, embarrassing, or humorous, that's at least better to look back on than a horrible first time.

More often than not, these were the stories that were openly told in the presence of others with the speaker sometimes gathering people around saying, "You've got to hear this one." Occasionally they would even open with, "I love telling this story."

There's a "better them than me" element to the stories in this section. Ridiculous or embarrassing as they were, at least it made these entries memorable, unique and most everyone was able to laugh about them now.

ANOTHER NOTCH ON THE BEDPOST
Chris, 22

I grew up in a really small town, graduating class of 70 people. Real small farm town, very church-oriented, Christian-oriented so I had a very sheltered life growing up. My parents wouldn't let me have girls over without keeping the door completely wide open.

I graduated from high school a virgin and I got a summer job working for the highway department and worked with a girl who was home for summer from college. She had her own apartment in a town nearby and while my parents thought I was going to work, I would call In sick and we'd hang at her place. We hung out for about a week, then one night we were partying and I didn't really get drunk at the time but she got drunk and pulled me into her bedroom. We started making out and I didn't really want to do anything, I was so scared 'cause I was still a virgin. She just grabbed me and stuck me inside of her. So she just kind of broke me. That was it.

The next night I go over to her apartment, walk up the stairs and when I open the door she's got about six drunk friends with her and when they see me they all start chanting, "21, 21, 21!" I hung out long enough to find out that she had just broke up with her longtime college boyfriend of two years, moved home, and I was the 21st guy she had been with in a month. I was pretty embarrassed.

The next night I met number 19 or 20, 'cause he came by to see her. It made me feel kind of bad when I saw one of the guys she slept with right before me because he looked like a cracked out drug addict. It definitely brought sex in a whole new light for me. At that age I was still a young kid who never drank, never partied, never did anything. I had this ideal about sex, especially being brought up in the church. That ideal was snapped away from me. Made me realize that sex wasn't that big of a deal.

I pretty much stopped talking to her a week after that so I never found out what her final number was. But I do know that about a year after that she got engaged to a guy and got married after dating him for only six or seven months. After having one guy for so long then breaking up, she went crazy and then got serious with a guy again. I happened to meet her during the crazy part.

> She had obviously lost her virginity before because while we were having sex she said I was better than any Italian she ever had.
>
> *Thomas, 38*
> *Amarillo, Texas*

(...and how not to)

I WANT TO BE INSIDE OF YOU, STAT
Alan, 37

It was with my high school sweetheart. We started dating when I was 15 and I was totally guilt-ridden about sex. All we would do was make out, but we'd make out for hours and hours and I'm still trying to find a girl who can kiss as well as she can.

We're making out and she slid her hand down my pants. Suddenly I'm thinking, "Wait a minute, it's OK?" It opened up the flood gates and I was constantly pestering her. We fooled around like that all the time leading up to the moment I actually lost my virginity, which was in my grandmother's house.

My grandmother was away visiting my aunt and we lied to my girlfriend's parents and said we were going to see *The Last Dragon*. It's like this Motown martial arts movie starring Vanity. I've never seen it, but to this day it still means something to me.

We have to go through the basement to get inside my grandmother's house. We go inside and we go to one of the spare rooms. So I got this condom, I'm at least that prepared, and my grandmother was a nurse so I find this lubricant for surgical instruments. I'm thinking, "That's safe. You can put that inside."

So we're using that for lube and I'm trying to be gentle 'cause I want to be invited back, you know. And she's like, "It's burning! It's burning!" Apparently the surgical cream was not a good sex lube. So we stop and we start again. I actually did eventually get inside of her but I thought it was rude to do any thrusting so I kind of just laid on top of her. She didn't move either, it was just one person laying on top of another person for about an hour

Afterwards we were sitting there waiting for a moment and we're both trying to say something significant. She's like, "So, do you feel different." I'm like, "No."

We ended up going out for six years.

...IN YOUR MOUTH, NOT IN YOUR HAND
Gabriel, 28

Me and my high school girl were laying in my bed eating M&M's. We ended up doing the business. Afterwards we're laying around chillin'. I get up to move and I see this big fuckin' brown stain on the sheets. Then I saw the look on her face and I think, "Aw, fuck man. I know I wiped!" I look closer and I see some green bits in there and I'm like, "What the fuck?" So I get down there and I smell it, "Wait, that ain't shit." I taste it – it's chocolate. I notice the M&M's bag. They had rolled out of the bag and our body heat must have melted them in my sheets. So I said, "Look baby. This is M&M's." You know, I'm all clean and cool. Once I proved it was chocolate we were all happy again.

DO YOU HAVE ANYTHING TO DECLARE?
Bill W, 27

SHAWN WICKENS: Alright, so tell me about where it happened.

BILL W: So I was in London... with my buddy Mike here. We were there on vacation, whatever. And we got in tight... we became friendly with a couple of the bartenders at our hotel. One of them, her name was Andrea; we were hanging out with them. One night we went back with them to their place and Andrea had the adjoining room. And... I lost my virginity, and then about four weeks later I found that I had crabs.

SW: You didn't see her again after you found out you had crabs?

BW: I had come back to the states by then. We were only In London for about a week. So this was a couple weeks later.

SW: Oh. You came back with the European crabs.

BW: Yes, exactly so...

SW: So was that a story that came out immediately amongst all of your friends?

BW: Pretty much. It's been spread around. My fiancé knows about it.

SW: Had that deterred you from hooking up with random chicks?

BW: Absolutely. No more... that was my first and last one-night stand. That's it.

MIKE: You missed the whole part of the story. He's not good at telling stories.

BW: OK. As a postscript, in order to get it taken care of. I had to ask my mother for health insurance, so I wound up having to tell her about the whole tale of woe, which her first response was, "You fucking idiot."

SW: Did you try getting rid of them on your own before going to her?

BW: I went to one of those first-med places and they gave me some prescription and it didn't work that well. So I ended up having to go to an actual dermatologist to get it taken care of. After a week they were gone. I think my friends probably would tell the story better.

M: Then he told the rest of us. We were getting stoned one night, I didn't realize he had gotten crabs. I had went with him to London. And we were in a park... a playground of our old elementary school. Me and about seven other friends, and we were a little high, maybe a little drunk, and he said, "Oh yeah, by the way everybody. I got crabs." Yeah, everyone knows.

(...and how not to)

GLAD THAT'S OUT OF THE WAY
Gina, 23

My boyfriend and I had a history of embarrassing physical encounters. The first time we kissed or anything was after the prom our freshman year of high school. We all slept over at a friend's house, five couples with blankets and everything all over the floor. We were making out and he was on top of me and then he just suddenly stopped and rolled off of me like he was going to go to sleep. I thought it meant I was a bad kisser because he just completely ignored me. He went to the bathroom, came back, and went to sleep without saying anything.

A couple weeks later, I found out from the baseball team that he had jizzed his pants from making out and was embarrassed to tell me about it. He wasn't too embarrassed to tell his baseball team though, so they gave him the nickname Quick Draw McGraw.

We were finally ready to have sex in the tenth grade. We were in the back of his pickup truck, and of course it was painful. Then he went down on me and said I was really wet. He comes up and had blood all over his face. I didn't want to say anything, it was that bad. He saw himself in the rearview mirror and he was pretty cool about it. I mean we lost our virginity at the same time so it was something we went through together. After that the hymen was broke, no more blood to worry about.

> "What I remember most about it was that outside her window was a famous house by Frank Lloyd Wright called the Robie House. I can remember after having sex laying on the bed and looking out the window at the Robie House and feeling, "Wow. That really is an amazing piece of architecture."
> *Edward, 28*
> *Chicago, Illinois*

OOPS. MY BAD
T.J., 26

She was 16, I was 16, and after four months of going out she consented and we decided to have sex.

She had to have a hip operation after a car accident when she was younger and she threw her hip out the first time we were doing it. There was a lot of screaming from her end which cut everything off. That didn't steer me away from sex though. There's certain human instincts that override that kind of initial trauma.

HOW ROMANTIC
Scott, 24

The loss of virginity took place in the Lower East Side in New York City, in the St. Mark's Hotel, during high school, eight or nine years ago. What's interesting about the St. Mark's Hotel is that they have an hourly rate. Normally I think it's about $45 an hour, but for two hours it was $75, so we opted for the two hours.

I had met my girlfriend through a mutual friend in high school – Bronx Science. She was one of my close friend's ex-girlfriends, oddly enough. He introduced me to her at his party and that's where we met.

We dated for about a year and a half and she felt like she was too young at that point and of course I supported that decision. She was about 14 and I was very young too, just a couple months older than her. So there was a whole courting period for a year and a half and she refused to lose her virginity before she was 16. When I got to be 16, my friends were all bragging about getting it and they were 15. I had been with the same girl since I was 15 so my hormones were raging.

Weeks after she turned 16, I started pestering her again and again, "You know you're 16 now. You don't want to be a hypocrite." That went on for a couple of weeks. Eventually it was our actual anniversary, our year and a half anniversary 'cause we were at that age when you celebrate six-month anniversaries, which is not really an anniversary, I know, but everything aligned perfectly.

I took her to the St. Mark's Hotel; I think it was a Thursday. At the time I worked at Credit Suisse First Boston doing fax running jobs. A fax would come in, I would take the fax and drop it off to a banker. It was like nine bucks an hour so I put about 10 hours of pay into the afternoon.

When we walked inside the hotel I was shocked that they gave us the room because we didn't have any ID. We hadn't even bothered getting fakes. We just said that we needed two hours and the guy led us in and he turned on the television, this old 13" television with the rotary dials, turned it on to hardcore porno, walked out and closed the door behind him. It was a very surreal way to start out.

The room, I'd say, was about 10 x 8. The bathroom was outside in the hallway. It was just like totally rundown. The window blinds were the kind where you could still kind of see outside so we were trying to close those as much as possible. Even though the St. Mark's Hotel doesn't look out onto the street, we were very much interested in feeling as protected as possible.

There were no blankets, no sheets on the bed. There was a bed spread and nothing else. That really bugged her so I had to go out and demand sheets, which was an odd thing to go through. And she refused to have the TV left on.

At the end of the night we lost track of time. Of course it wasn't two hours of blissful losing of virginity. It was mostly like an hour and a half of awkwardness leading up to it. Then doing it was 30 more minutes of awkwardness. But we totally lost track of time and the management started banging on the door at the end of the two hours. We started freaking out because for whatever reason we assumed we could get arrested for doing what we were doing. There was no reasoning behind it. But it was like a bunch of kids trying to hide their drugs, like we were just running around trying to get dressed while this guy was constantly banging and we were like, "OK. We're coming. We're coming." But he didn't stop; nonstop banging. So that was a wonderful way to usher in a new level of maturity.

(...and how not to)

HOME RUN ON THE THIRD SWING
Christian, 24

I went to a party with my friends who were a little bit older than me. They were going into their freshman year and I was going into my seventh grade year. We went to a party and we were playing "spin the bottle," which turned into "seven minutes in heaven."

My first spin landed on a girl. We kissed. I spun it a second time and it landed on her again so we had to make out. Then on my third turn it happened again and everyone was like, "You guys gotta do something. You gotta go in the closet," because it landed on her three times in a row. It was just the luck of the draw, and there were like eight people down in that basement.

My buddies were calling me scared and making fun of me, so I had to go through with it. We ended up having sex in the closet. It was dark in there. I was just going along with it. So we had sex for pretty much like 45 seconds and then I came out smiling like, "Yeah." And my buddies were asking, "So what did you guys do?" I'm all smiling, "Yeah, it was great." She came out adjusting her clothes and she says, "He was a 'less than a minute-man'." It was a really bad situation because everyone made fun of me. But either way, I would have lost. They would have made fun of me if I didn't go in there. Then when I did go in there, I still got made fun of.

Then she found out I was still only in the sixth grade, going into seventh, and then everyone made fun of her so I got her back in a way.

So... it could have been better but I still had a great time.

PUBERTY... IT'S HARD
Aaron, 37

It was with my high school sweetheart and I know that's such a chemically charged saying but that's what she was, my sweetheart. I'm from Modesto, California, and it was about 108 degrees one summer day, but we had decided that was the day. Her parents were gone; we planned on meeting at her place. This was discussed over the phone and through her bedroom window the night before. You know, real classy.

Physically there was some strange stuff going on like, "No, no, no, no, yes." Then "Pop!" it was over. We both walked back to my house in a daze.

I have kind of a pigeon chest that I'm really kind of shy about so I kept on this white T-shirt when we did it. I didn't notice until it was too late but that white shirt had a big arrow of blood that went from my crotch up to my shoulders. Real fine lines of blood like almost in a perfect 'V' pointed down right at my crotch. We didn't know it was there until we walked into to my house my mom went, "Oh my god! What the hell happened to you?!"

I probably told her I fell off my bike. We were in such shock that I was covered in evidence.

ZAPPED!
Vance M, 23

VANCE M: It was with this girl... Cameron. I don't remember how I knew her. She lived about 30 minutes away, in a different town, from where I grew up in Columbus, Ohio. I think I met her at like a swimming pool when I was 13 or something like that. The only other time I ever hung out with her was when I went over to her mom's house once and it was the first time I ever watched *Cheech and Chong's Up in Smoke*.

SHAWN WICKENS: That's a life-changing movie.

VM: Yeah. But I didn't smoke pot. Then it was near the end of eighth grade. And... it was in the summer and she actually invited me to some party out on some land, in her town, which was a few towns over. I went out there and I remember we walked off into the woods a little bit. We were kissing and then it started inevitably leading towards that. And... I remember we had started having sex and about five seconds into it and I just decided I didn't want to. And I just got this bad panic and anxiety and I thought, "What the fuck am I doing? I don't even... I don't *know* this girl." It was just like this overwhelming thing of a girl asking me to have sex and I was like, "I guess I say yes."

Friend: Was she older?

VM: I wish. No. I think she was my age. I think the reason I said yes was because I just didn't know. Like what else do you say when a girl asks you to have sex? But, five seconds into it I made up some excuse like, "Oh I think... the condom is hurting me. This condom's too small. I think it's cutting off my circulation," or something like that. But I made up some really bad excuse and said, "I'm gonna... I'm gonna go." And then like I started walking off and she got up to follow me and then I heard her scream. She had walked right into an electric fence.

SW: Wow... how did you avoid it?

VM: I don't remember. I think I was somehow... I was lucky enough to avoid it. At that point God stepped in and kept her away from me. And I remember I just like, I heard it and I asked, "Are you all right?" She was like, "I think so." And then I just kept walking... I was freaked out. I wanted to get out of there.

SW: You were freaked out about who you were having sex with or you were freaked out about the sex?

(...and how not to)

VM: I think it was a bit of both. The idea of it was something I was more fixated on then the actual act. And once I was in the moment it was, "I don't want this." This was always something that has been dangled over your head, especially as a male. Growing up, it's something you are meant to pursue always and it's like the ultimate goal of any interaction with a female. And it was a good lesson because I finally realized this was not the definite end of the road that I wanted to pursue. This is just something that's there. And I think I just had that realization and went about backing out of it in a very bad way. We never spoke again. And that was pretty much it.

SW: And how did you get home?

VM: My stepfather came and picked me up later on in the evening.

SW: You didn't see her at her place?

VM: It wasn't at her place it was at some friend's house. It was kind of out in the country and... I remember I actually ran off with one of her friends and like me and her buddy were hiding in the woods and like I could hear the girl wandering around and asking for me and I was like, "I don't want to talk to her. This is going to be too weird."

SW: You were like hiding in bushes or something?

VM: Yeah. Well it was kind of in the forest a little bit. We were hiding behind trees and stuff... That's all I got.

> I thought it would be funny to keep my shoes on. So I was completely naked, except for a pair of black socks and a pair of red Chuck Taylors. My gf didn't think it was funny when I told her I kept them on on purpose.
> *Jarvis, 24*
> *Annapolis, Maryland*

CLOSE CALL
Marky, 26

All my family was over for Christmas Eve. After dinner my girlfriend and I snuck up to my room and had sex. And luckily we were finished and had our clothes on when my mom came in looking for us. We were sitting on my couch, my mom sat down on the bed and the funniest part of the story was when, at one point, she leaned back and put her hand on the wet spot on the sheets my girlfriend had made, that had soaked through the comforter.

My girlfriend and I both saw it. I don't know how my mom couldn't have known. Or maybe she chose to be cool about it. I never asked her.

A NEW SENSATION
Kyle, 36

I reunited with this girl I had a crush on in middle school at a high school dance and we hit it off. We made a date. The interesting thing about it was that I only had my learner's permit and I was three months away from turning 16 and getting my real driver's license. She didn't know this and totally assumed that I could pick her up for our date. This was a problem because technically I couldn't drive by myself. Yet there's this woman that I'm interested in, or girl rather, who wants to go on a date. So... I stole my older brother's car.

He was back from college but he was off doing some stuff with his friends. My brother's 1986 Honda Accord was available and sitting in the driveway. Sweet, sweet ride – the sporty hatchback model and the keys were in his room. I lifted those and went on my first real date.

I took her to a movie and basically we were making out the whole time, which was a strange thing for me because this was not like my normal understanding of going to the movies. I actually wanted to watch *Beverly Hills Cop*. I was trying to pay attention, but the whole experience began with that whole tension between wanting to and not being all that comfortable making out in a public place.

And in my mind I was thinking, "OK, this is what the evening is going to be." Making out in the movie theater. That's the evening, that's the peak. And I was like, "That's beautiful. That's fantastic. I'm a happy man."

We got back into the car and she was like, "Why don't we go somewhere?" Now I'm thinking that the clock's ticking. I got to get this car back and at the same time my parents don't know that I'm out and about and that's also going to be a problem. On top of all of that, where are we gonna go? This was in San Antonio and in San Antonio at that time there really wasn't any place for kids to go hang out. You could go to a McDonald's or something like that but there were no real cool places to go. She says, "There's a park nearby. We could go hang out there." "OK, good idea." I'm still not even thinking that something more was going to happen.

We drive to the park and she's all, "Oh, over here is a place where we can be alone for awhile." "OK, great. Sure." But the safety factor is getting to be more and more dire. The window is closing, now it's probably about 11:30 at night.

We're now both sitting in the front seat of the car, just talking and I could tell there's some sort of tension going on but I'm trying to make amusing conversation, which is apparently not very amusing. I'm trying to talk about the movie that we didn't even get to watch and eventually I just realized that maybe we could make out again and, gee... wouldn't that'd be great? So I moved in and we started making out and things got a little bit more heated. We're pawing at clothes, feeling each other up, and the kissing got rough.

Then she starts pulling me over the gear shift, it was an automatic, so I maneuver over and now we're both in the passenger seat. Things are getting more frisky and she takes her top off. I'm thinking, "What? This is fantastic." I'm loving it. Things keep going more and more in that direction and eventually I'm like, "Hey... I might have a shot at this. I might actually be able to do this." I didn't know exactly what to do, but I was very enthusiastic about it.

(...and how not to)

    I had some trouble with her belt buckle, finally got that off. And what added to the tension too was that there was a very palpable perception on her part, albeit an inaccurate one, that I knew what I was doing and that it was maybe the entire reason for us being out that night. I was a reasonably obnoxious young man and I had a lot of confidence just not necessarily in that arena. So maybe that and some of her past experiences led her to the conclusion that I had been around. I technically and anatomically knew what was supposed to happen, but I'd never been in that position before and certainly not in the front bucket seat of a very cramped Honda Accord. And a stolen Honda Accord at that. Well it gets worse.

    One thing did lead to another. We figured out how "tab A" fit with "slot B" without much difficulty. The problem occurred when things started moving, things were going along and I'm feeling a relatively new sensation and trying to move and suddenly I'm completely overcome with worry. Worry that I'm not going to be able to perform this action properly, worried that while she was making very nice noises they seemed to me a little fake, a little disingenuous. A little like she was encouraging me by making those noises rather than her genuinely feeling those noises. And I have no idea, where to put my hands, no idea if I should be kissing her, you know, what should I be doing? And at that exact moment when I'm getting excited, and I can feel it, I get the guilt that comes from thinking, "I'm getting close and this could be a really great thing but I don't know if she's close." At that moment I kicked the air conditioning hose loose from underneath the dashboard on the passenger's side. So now I don't know what I'm doing, I'm struggling with the mere concept that I'm doing this in a stolen car that I've now apparently destroyed, and there's ice cold water pouring over my feet.

    I didn't immediately know what I broke which added to the confusion of the whole ordeal, but I knew that I had damaged the car and everything in my brain was telling me, "This is not right. This must end. This has to stop," so I did. Technically I view it as losing my virginity because there was intercourse even though I didn't actually come to climax. And I'm pretty damn certain that she didn't either. It was a very sloppy, inarticulate, not well done, "OK, I'll take you home now" kind of experience.

    I dropped her off knowing that this was definitely not what she anticipated and knowing full well that I was probably never going to see her again. Our one abortive little attempt at it was an indication to her that it would all be bad, all wrong, all stupid. There was no kiss good night, there was a, "OK. Well I'll see you later, I guess..."

    I drove home and immediately parked the car and tried to figure out what the hell was going on with it, had no idea. Replaced the keys, got into bed as quickly as I possibly could, and pulled the covers up to my chin.

    I woke up the next morning to hear my dad and brother talking about it and my dad saying, "Well, you know... Hondas do that. There's a loose fitting on Hondas and so it must have hit a pothole or something and broke loose." My dad just figured that the hose had, "Come loose... somehow". To this day I'm certain that my brother has no idea that I was the 'cause. But I'm pretty sure that my mother knows something.

The mysterious hose problem was all that they talked about that night over dinner conversation too. My father saying, "Well I heard Hondas have problems with those things." And my brother saying, "We put it back on easily enough so it must have just come loose on its own." My mom wasn't saying a thing, but looking right at me. She was just staring. So I'm pretty sure she suspected I was somehow to blame.

I never did see that girl again. And it wasn't for not looking. I did keep an eye out for her at football games whenever our two high schools were playing or relative times when people that I knew from my middle school were around. I would ask, "Hey, what's happening with Miranda?" Nobody ever knew... she disappeared on me.

> This girl lived down the street from me and she seduced me. Two years later my mom and her dad start dating and then they get married. So I see this girl at the wedding and it's like, "What's up? I guess you're my stepsister now." I never really see her anymore.
>
> *Garvin, 22*
> *Salt Lake City, Utah*

I WAS ROBBED!
Shandra, 22

I'm from Metairie, just about 7 minutes from New Orleans. I met the guy over a phone conversation, I was 13 years old. My friend had met him and the three of us were kind of like talking on the same call... three-way call. I think she saw him and they weren't attracted to each other but he still got her number probably to meet some of her other 13-year-old friends. The three of us were talking and she decided that she didn't like him so she hung up and he and I talked about him coming over.

He came over that afternoon and we were kissing. This is like my first thing of everything, like I'd never made out with a boy, no one ever felt my breasts or my cootchie before. We just did a whole fucking grand slam.

He was 17, I was 13. For a condom we used a Ziploc bag. Oh my god, it hurt! We had sex and after he left I found out he stole like 50 bucks from me. I was making part-time money working at a city playground concession stand for three dollars an hour selling popcorn, candy and drinks, and ICEEs and stuff. After he left I looked in my little smiley face, little zip-up purse and saw it was gone. And he took a picture of me too. I took that as a compliment because then he had something to remember me by, but not the money part. It felt like I paid to lose my virginity. Supposedly he was in a gang, The Bloods, you know like gangster or whatever.

My dad came home about an hour after he left so it was kind of weird. Thank God he didn't come home while we were having sex on the couch... 'cause we had sex at least like 20 times... 'cause I was so tight. I was a tight, little virgin. But I didn't bleed. My cherry has never been popped apparently 'cause I never bled.

(...and how not to)

NOT A LESBIAN
Leslie, 24

This happened with a 21-year-old letch of a guy who lived on this one street in Des Moines that my friends and I called "CrackDonald's" because people would drive through there and buy crack. Yeah, this guy was really going places. I was 16 and I was a lifeguard. I was really fit and really tan, but tan in a way that it looked like I was wearing a pale, white one-piece swimsuit. This guy totally seduced me. We were smoking pot and watching cartoons and it turned into, you know, "Roman hands and Russian fingers" then five minutes later I wasn't wearing any clothes. I did have my swimsuit that day because I just got done from work so he got to get a good eyeful of that first. Plus I smelled of chlorine and sunscreen – sexy. And he smelled of pot and b.o. – real sexy.

So it was on the floor where his roommate... God this is so disgusting, where one of his roommates always slept. Like ten people lived there, it was sort of a hippie house. The whole time I was losing my virginity, a roommate was pounding on the windows with his shoe trying to break in because he had lost his keys and I guess he had something important to do. It wasn't very romantic. When we got done I said, "My curfew is midnight, gotta go."

So the whole thing lasted maybe 20 minutes. Thinking about it makes me shudder. He didn't even take off his shirt and his junkie roommate was pounding on the window the whole time.

I met the letch through another job. I was a bus girl at a place called the Drake Diner. He was a waiter and we met rolling silverware and I was totally in love with him. He did well at that diner, he later on got a blow job from our 28-year-old manager in the restaurant office.

Then, check this out, he dumped me by telling me that he cheated on me. But here's the kicker, not only did he cheat on me... he cheated on me with four people at the exact same time. I'm like, "You know if you're going to have a wild sexy orgy you can at least invite me." He was just a big ol' ding-dong.

Now he's fat and has a child and lives in Iowa City where he's still a letch. My best friend from back home called me up not long ago and said the letch tried to pick her up in a bar.

But in spite of all of that, I had fun. I was happy to take sex off my to-do list. And I was happy to find out that sex was fun and that I wasn't a lesbian.

> This girl said to me, "I want you to go down on me first." I was like, "OK, I'll go for it," and pardon my French but her pussy stunk so bad – so, so bad. It was dark so what I did was I tried to make like a mouth with my hand and use that on her while I made slurping noises with my mouth.
>
> *Clyde, 33*
> *Tulsa, Oklahoma*

How to Lose Your Virginity

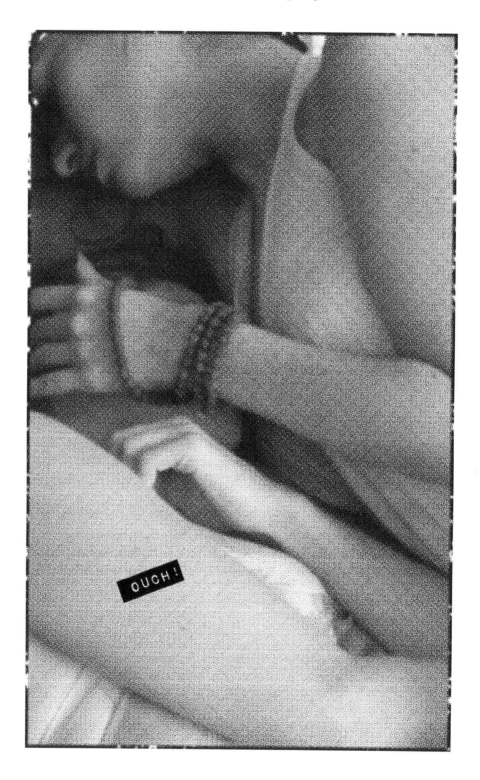

(...and how not to)

"WE DROP-KICKED OUR CHERRIES."

9

Regret. "What have I done?" "How could I have been so stupid?" "Why did I waste it on him?" "I can't believe I slept with her."

First impressions are a bitch. A rough first day at a new school can taint the rest of one's academic career. A bad first day at a new job can affect how new coworkers look upon you for weeks, even months. Depending on the severity of the first impression, it can take a lot of effort to recover and reverse the damage. And a bad first time can drive one towards a jaded outlook of sex for years. So, it's fitting that a quote taken from this first story be used as the name for this chapter.

Sex-ed classes teach safe physical ways to have sex, yet as far as I can recall, safe emotional ways to have sex were never discussed. As one interviewee wisely stated, "If you're not comfortable talking about sex, you're not ready to have it." Sometimes you're not ready to have it even if you are comfortable with talking about it. Many of these males and females thought they were ready but in hindsight, wish they had held on a little longer.

OUCH
Diane, 25

Sixteen years old, with a guy I ultimately wasn't very attracted to. I hate to say it but my friend summed it up the best... "We drop-kicked our cherries." It's such a horrible way to put it, but it's true. And that's about how intimate it was. Me with one guy and her with another.

We both lost our virginity together, we were literally five feet away from each other in this one dude's basement.

Why him? Why then? I was 16 years old. I was impatient and idiotic. We were stupid. I didn't understand the full significance of it until a few months later. Somehow, some guy I actually liked found out and he gave me shit for it. He made fun of me for losing my virginity. It was tough.

> I probably told her at least 50 times that I didn't want to have sex. But I was drunk and horny and I wanted her to blow me and then she grabbed it and put it in. I was just tired of resisting and saying no.
>
> *Glen, 24*
> *Cleveland, Ohio*

THE JUSTIFICATION
James, 27

I was a senior, about to graduate from college. It was a week before I was going to turn 22 and I did not want to be a 22-year-old virgin. There was this freshman foreign exchange student from Russia with a real groovy accent and even though I didn't like her very much, I had been flirting with her for about two weeks. She had been out drinking one night and she came to my room and knocked on my door and said, "Get a sleeping bag and take me to the TV station." I worked at the college TV station so I had keys and I spent so much of my four years there so it was kind of a special place. She knew I wanted to do it there. The TV station had a couch and we wouldn't have to worry about my roommate around so that's where we went.

I should have said no. We didn't have a condom and she told me before we did it to make sure she didn't get pregnant. Like, "OK, I'll do what I can."

We had sex, she wanted to do it again but I didn't. So she got mad and left. And it's good that she did because later that morning the fire marshall was going around checking fire extinguishers. He unlocked the door and walked in on me sleeping on the couch. He could have walked in on both of us naked.

The way I look at it, I abandoned my principles because I had told myself that I wouldn't have sex with a woman who didn't mean anything to me. But I did hold on to my ethics because I never told her I loved her. In fact I told her I didn't love her and there couldn't be anything between us and she still wanted to fuck. She claimed I was her first, but later on I heard rumors that she was rampantly bisexual and had been with all kinds of girls but no guys. I don't know.

It was really dumb and it made the next time, when it was with someone I actually did care about, it made that next time less significant than it could have been.

(...and how not to)

A DISSERVICE TO WOMEN EVERYWHERE
Patricia, 42

I was 14 in 1976. 1976 was a big year – the bicentennial. My parents were divorced and I had a big falling out with my father. So in an act of rebellion I started going out with a guy my father did not approve of.

This guy, Trey, had a beard, he worked in an auto body shop, I mean he was not the cream of the crop. He drove a dark green, MG convertible and he could buy beer and pot and so we were sort of an item for the most of the summer of '76 and the months beyond.

I guess I was in the mood to do something drastic because it happened Christmas Eve and after Christmas Eve dinner ended I went over to my best friend's house who lived two doors away. Trey and my friend and this other guy were over there and there was no denying that sex was in the air. Of course we ending up smoking pot and drinking some beer but then someone put on Rod Stewart's song "Tonight's the Night," so the mood was engineered by these two guys.

We went into this other room and he and I had made out before, but I had never gone all the way. I didn't really know what "all the way" was. So while we had kissed before, we had never really gotten that physical. That night I felt moved in that direction; compelled to do it since the clothes had come off and my friend was doing it in the next room.

It was a very unsatisfying experience. I was so shocked. I thought for sure that this man, who was 20, would know what to do. I think he was drunk and nervous, in that order, but he couldn't keep hard like Kyle MacLachlan in *Sex and the City* – he could raise his sails but he couldn't get it into the harbor.

I was menstruating and as a 14-year-old you're kind of new to menstruating and as far as sex goes, I didn't really know that I could move around. I never heard from him again. I asked my best girlfriend, "Why is he gone, what happened?" She said that Trey had told her that he didn't want to fuck a log. Of course he was fucking a log, I was 14, I was menstruating, I was lying to my parents so I could have sex with my older boyfriend in a basement. I was just so freaked out about everything I really didn't know what to do.

I was so thoroughly disappointed and shocked by his unpleasant and callous treatment and it did two things to me. It made me want to become the best lover ever and I've made quite a bit of progress on that score. And it also made me lose about a hundred points of respect for all men. There was such a lack of compassion and sensitivity and instruction even, on his part. I mean you gotta know that if you're doing a virgin you're going to need to tell her a thing or two.

I saw him a few years later when I was 17. I was just about to graduate from high school and I had gotten an early decision at a few universities, had done very well. I had my driver's license and really had my act together. He walked over with a big smile and tried to start some small-talk conversation. I looked at him dead in the eye and was very curt and didn't let him off the hook because if you deflower a virgin you really have a bit of an obligation to ease her into that new life, because her life is never going to be the same again. He didn't do that and I look at it as a betrayal to the art of sex, which really can be quite beautiful and expressive and to do that to me, a sweet, nice looking, smart girl from a good family... it was just really pathetic on his part. I only credit the years and years of counseling that I've been able to endure that allows me to not hold it against every man I've ever been with.

IT'S A SIN TO KILL A MOCKINGBIRD
Alexandra C, 31

ALEXANDRA C: It happened on a snow day. A snow day when I was in the eighth grade. I was 13.

SHAWN WICKENS: Where are you from?

AC: Originally I'm from Michigan. And I had moved down here to Nashville and it was with a boy from my math class. And um...

SW: How did the day begin?

AC: I found out it was a snow day because I'm an insomniac and I was up all night watching it snow. And when I realized I didn't have to go to school the next day the first thing on my mind was, "Well, I get to be alone with this boy," because he lived down the street. And he skated over.

SW: You called him?

AC: Of course. And I guess we both kind of knew what everything was going to lead up to and it did. And it wasn't fantastic, and it wasn't mind-blowing and it wasn't what I had expected it to be at all. It was just this thing that happened and it felt strangely adult.

SW: Did you guys discuss, did you have an adult conversation?

AC: We had a conversation in the only way that we knew how, I think, which was... I think I was kind of crying afterward and I said that I felt funny about it. I felt bad in my stomach after I had it.
My best friend was older and she had had sex with someone and I think she lied and said it was great and wonderful and then when I went ahead and did it, I realized the gravity of what had happened. Being the only girl in my class who had that kind of knowledge when kids were still making out and feeling over the shirt... I had had intercourse and that was extraordinarily disturbing to me on many levels.

SW: Did anybody find out?

AC: That's... silly you should say that because my group of friends had perceived me to be the girl that you went to to find out about things because I was experienced and that wasn't necessarily the case. I mean the whole thing turned me into a serial monogamist. I didn't want to necessarily do this thing all the time with everyone I met. And I was terrified of it. And that's what people never understood.

SW: Did he make subsequent advances that you had to deny?

AC: The crux of our relationship became purely sexual, as much as sexuality between two extraordinarily young people can be. But yeah, sure and... we both did and we both, it was any time, any place, in a field, at school. Whatever. It just became the reason for being.

(...and how not to)

SW: That's probably all you understood relationships to be.

AC: I stayed up the entire night before reading *To Kill a Mockingbird*. All in one sitting. And... I think that's had more of a profound effect on me than the sex. Would I have waited if I could do it over? Probably. I think it's served only to turn me bitter and to expect much more out of people than they are able or willing to give.

SW: Had he read the book as well?

AC: No, he was not smart. He was cute, but he wasn't smart.

SW: No literary conversations then?

AC: No. No, God... Jesus. no. For most of the time when I was in junior high and later in high school I only had sex with people I could dominate. It's true. Because that's what I perceived the act to be about. There wasn't love involved, there was me telling boys or making boys do what I wanted them to do. And then in the end, they got off. I didn't, but it certainly made me happy to manipulate people.

    I didn't get off my first time but he did and that's... I guess, in the end, that's what was important to me – that the guy got off. And I felt better for making that happen for someone. Sick, co-dependent, passive-aggressive. Whatever you want to call it, that's how it was.

SW: Well if you couldn't get off you were the cause of... you made somebody else feel good.

AC: Exactly. I was the catalyst for someone else's good feeling. And that was enough. It wasn't until I was married until I thought that I had something close to meaningful sex.

> I went downstairs and the girl who was dating my brother asked me, "Did you just have sex with Billy?" I was like, "Yeah." And she said, "Ohmigod. You look exactly like you did before you two went upstairs." My hair was the same, there was no makeup taken off my face – nothing was different. And my brother was so mad because I had sex on his bed and with his best friend.
>
> *Marisa, 22*
> *Pottsville, Pennsylvania*

RACE RELATIONS
Will, 27

My assistant manager at the United Artists theater I worked at was all into me and I didn't want him at all, we were just friends. Brandon was black and, not that there is anything wrong with that, but it ultimately becomes important to the story.

Anyways, I was driving him home one night after work and he was talking real dirty. He was well hung and I could totally see it in his pants. I had lied to him before, because I didn't want to sound like a virgin and had said that I had sex before when I was in high school, even though I had not. I really lost it that night when I was 20 years old.

So he was under the impression I had sex before and he was telling me, "I've never had sex. I wanna have a first time. You're my friend, let me have sex with you." I was like, "I don't wanna have sex with you. I hate you."

I'm driving around and we're near my house, which is off this road with all these brand-new housing developments. There were all these paved roads with nothing on them so finally after all his constant nagging I was like, "Fine. Is that all you fucking want?" I was pissed and annoyed so I turned off the road and we stopped at a dark, little cul-de-sac. I turn off the car and I was like, "Fine. Take out your fucking dick." He takes it out and it's huge, I'm like, "Good fucking Lord." It's so huge, I didn't know what to do with it.

We start with making out but when Brandon makes out he wraps his lips completely around your mouth and he's like inhaling your face. So by the time I'm done making out with him my whole face was like dripping with saliva. Already I was mortified. Then I realize I have to go down on him. I've already gone this far and it's what he's expecting. I go down there and it's so big I swear to God after a minute and a half my jaw was aching. I was hurting and I couldn't go too far down 'cause I started choking. He's not finishing and I'm doing it forever. It's not phasing him at all and I need to breathe so we stop.

I decided let's just go in the backseat and give each other a rest. We go back there and you know he wants me to do it some more to him, so I'm like, "Oh, fucking hell." I start doing it some more and finally I'm just like, "You know why don't you go ahead and just try to do it to me." And I had never had a blow job so I had no idea what to expect. This was my first time for everything and I have to pretend I'm a seasoned veteran.

He puts his mouth on my penis and I swear to God five seconds later I'm coming. So he's like, "Do you always come this fast?" I'm like. "No, um... I was just really excited." I'm all embarrassed and it's like, "Oh shit. Now I've gotta make him come." So I'm working, working, working. Finally after forever he's like, "I don't know why I can't come." So he wants to like rub it on me. I'm like, "All right do whatever you gotta do." I'm laying there, and he's rubbing his penis all over my stomach.

We were doing it forever and I got hard again so I actually came again. He's still rubbing and finally he comes and I'm like, "Thank God." I used his shirt to clean everything up. I took him home and I just remember I was so horrified. I told him, "Don't tell anybody we did this," because we had all the same work friends. I was so embarrassed.

(...and how not to)

    I got home and, here's where the black part comes in. You know some black people have to keep their body lotioned up because their skin gets ashy. He always used this like cocoa butter crap on his body. So I get home, I get into bed and I'm reeking like cocoa butter and I'm feeling sticky all over because he was sweating and it dripped off on me. At this time I still lived with my parents. I didn't want to like take a shower at two in the morning and wake everybody up so I had to sleep all night smelling like cocoa butter. Oh, it was fucking horrible.

    I had to wash my sheets. I lied and told my mother that I took a shower and put my wet towel on my bed and so my sheets got all wet. I ended up moving out of my parents' house a week later.

    Then what happened afterwards is that Brandon was such a big mouth and he told my friend Mary Jane and I had to basically lie and tell him in front of Mary Jane, "Don't fucking lie," because it was horrible for me. I just didn't want anyone to know. He got really mad and offended by that, obviously, so we stopped talking.

THE ULTIMATUM
Steve, 28

New Year's Eve and my girl's parents were out of town. I'm not sure if there was a no-boys rule or anything but she threw a party with me, her, her friend, and my friend. I wasn't really into drinking then but I started boozing and smoking pot and that made her angry. But it was New Year's. What else do you do but get smashed? I grabbed a bottle of something out of her dad's liquor stash, lifted the bottle and took a drink and she was like, "No... don't. I'll give it up," and she handed me a condom. I was 15, she was 13 and her way to get me to not smoke or drink was to have sex with me.

    My friend was already off in another room doing it with my girlfriend's friend. I gave my girlfriend head for 30 minutes but I'm not sure if she came or not. After I gave her head we had sex for about, maybe 15 minutes.

    We did it, the act is done. I come out of the room and my buddy is finishing up and his girl is sitting there digging inside herself because the condom fell off inside of her and she already had a tampon inside her too. After they worked that out, my buddy and I left. It didn't keep me off drugs, I started doing stuff right after that.

    She was a sweet girl. I don't regret it but we were really young, I guess. It's led me down a weird path because now I'm pretty much open to sleeping with a lot of different people.

    I ran into her about a year ago and she didn't recognize me. That really hurt my feelings because this was the girl I lost my virginity to. I waved at her and she didn't even know who I was. It made me feel kind of bad because it was like a role reversal of things. Like guys are supposed to be the hard-asses.

THIS OTHER TIME, AT JOB CORPS...
Ruby, 24

I was 19 when I lost my virginity and I really wished I hadn't done it because I lost my virginity to a boy, who will remain nameless and I only did it because at the time I thought I didn't really need my virginity anymore. I was in Job Corps in Kentucky. It was a closed campus so you couldn't go anywhere off the campus grounds.

I lost it my second or third week there on Valentine's Day, right after the Valentine's Day dance. I had just broken up with a boyfriend specifically so I could go out with this other boy. Relationships at Job Corps are really, really messed up because you're with a person not quite 24 hours straight but you're with them a lot. The only time you're not interacting with them is during classes, unless you have classes together, and when you're sleeping. Pretty much the rest of the time you're with them constantly, so relationships can degenerate really, really quickly. I guess I was just horny and I was in the mood and I ended up losing it outside, behind a cafeteria. I was really embarrassed afterwards and I dumped that dude a couple days later.

But yeah, I lost my virginity in Job Corps like I'm sure several people have. And it was on Valentine's Day, you can't get any cheesier than that. He was a good ol' boy, country as all heck. Me being a country girl, he reminded me a lot about home. Job Corps was the first time I'd ever really been away from home so I'm sure there was a little bit of homesickness wrapped up in there.

Previous to this I lived a sheltered life when it came to guys. I knew what sex was and I knew it would happen some day. It wasn't the ideal time but I didn't force myself into the situation. It was just that I decided why not and I grabbed the first warm body that came my way.

He had great eyes and an endearing way that he held himself, this goofy, fun kind of a personality. His demeanor was more what I was focusing on that prevented me from seeing his teeth. Now when I look at a picture of him he's got such terrible teeth that stand out, the absolute worst teeth I've seen on a human being. And you can't see his personality in a picture, all you can see is his teeth. Nowadays I'm looking for better teeth.

My advice: If you haven't lost your virginity yet, and I'm not saying this for religious reasons or for social reasons, but if you haven't lost your virginity yet... wait. Wait, and I'm not saying wait until you're married but wait until you know it's going to be something special that you can remember. My memory is behind a cafeteria with my dress hitched up and my underwear around my ankles. You can't get any lamer than that when you're five feet away from a dumpster. Wait until there's a bed and candles and incense and it doesn't have to be true love, but there should be something between you and him that you'll remember forever.

If I could redo it, I would've waited and done it with this other guy who later on in the program became my best friend. George and I met the very first day I got to Job Corps. It was his first day also. He became a very, very good and trusted friend of mine and we left at the same time and we kept in touch and we remained friends all the way up until he was killed. He died in a car accident when a drunk driver hit him. I wish that I had lost it with George instead. I'm sure he knows. I still get little twinges and tickles from him that let me know he's around.

(see page 90)

(...and how not to)

HAVE YOU SEEN MY BROKEN HEART?
Melissa, 23

I was 17. I had just graduated high school. He was 23. We met through friends that I worked with. I was pretty experienced. I had just never had sex, but I was ready. I didn't love him or anything, I just thought it was time. So we fooled around for a couple of months and we finally did it on his living room floor. I still had my tennis shoes on.

It wasn't really a good experience because, as a girl, you build it up and you think your first time is supposed to be with someone you love. I wasn't even in a relationship with him. It was just a physical thing. I was scared and a little ashamed. Afterwards I went home and drank a bottle of cheap vodka and passed out.

The next morning I woke up and felt ashamed and felt like a different person. It was early and he called and I thought, "Oh, he cares. He's checking on me." Then he said, "Have you seen my wallet?" I thought, "This is not how this conversation is supposed to go."

I didn't tell anybody I lost my virginity for a week. I was so ashamed I couldn't even tell my best friend whom I normally went to for everything. The first person I went to was a male friend of mine and I was all upset because I didn't love the guy I had sex with. My friend said, "You know Melissa," and this made me feel better, "one day you will have sex with someone you love, and then your first time will really be irrelevant."

ADDICTED
Brett, 25

I was with my girlfriend of about two years. We went to see the Area: Two Festival with David Bowie, Moby and The Blue Man Group and I took some E for the second time in my life. I had taken it before with another friend of mine a while back but my girlfriend had never showed any interest in it. Then in the middle of the show she asked for some, which I feel bad about. I didn't force it on her, but it didn't feel right. And even though the sex felt real good, I'll never have sex on ecstasy ever again.

The actual experience itself was pretty good but we did it while we were on drugs and that's not the experience we were looking for. It didn't add anything. My first time was tainted. And never again did we ever do it drunk, or high, or on pills, or anything like that.

We were in a hotel after the show and it turned out she had her period so the sheets were bloody and we had to strip them off the bed. She was pretty bloody too so she had to shower. Our friends were next door and the next morning they told us they didn't get a wink of sleep. I didn't realize we were being loud because I was so out of it. But... the sex *was* pretty amazing and from then on I knew I'd be addicted... to the sex, that is.

SHHH... WE DON'T WANT TO WAKE UP MY EX-GIRLFRIEND
Jen, 27

I was 14 or 15, I was doing a bunch of drugs, you know, anything that was available and I ran away from home. Not the first time I ran away but the first time I ran away and meant it.

Harry Harwood was older and had an apartment. Just a guy I knew from exciting drug-crazed, fun and young, good times. I planned on living with him. That's where I imagined we'd end up, but... his ex-girlfriend was still at the apartment. They were broken up, she was sleeping in the bedroom and he was sleeping on the couch.

I was at his place and I had such a crush on him. We were making out on the living room floor and he turned to me and said, "So do you want to have sex?" I didn't know what to say so I replied, "What do you think?" We made out some more and then he started to push down on the top of my head. Obviously he wanted me to go down on him, but at the time I was all confused like, "Wait, I'm up here. Why are you pushing me down? We match right here by our faces."

I went down on him then we had sex and it was terrible and my head was banging into the coffee table the whole time. It didn't take long, maybe less than a minute and I remember him being very small. I didn't orgasm but, then again, I went into it knowing that wasn't going to happen. It was more about making him happy. I was just swept away by the excitement of leaving home and I was with this guy who had an apartment and he was an actor and that was all exciting. The sex didn't hurt so much. That was good. But my head hurt from banging against the coffee table, which probably took my mind off of any other pain. And Nine Inch Nails was playing in the background so whenever I hear *Pretty Hate Machine* I'm like, "Yep. My first time."

I was at least hoping it was going to be something special between us, but his ex-girlfriend was in the next room so how special is that? The next morning she told me I had to leave. On top of that, I was freaked out that we didn't use protection and I was sure I had AIDS because he had apparently been with everybody. I immediately got tested for everything but you have to wait because most STDs are dormant for several months so I got tested every six months for the next three years. I was so self-conscious about having sex with any boyfriend after that because I swore Harry Harwood gave me AIDS.

> I mean it probably happened. I would have done it if I was sober just because she was a willing, older girl. In retrospect I definitely should not have gotten that piss-drunk. In a weird, ridiculous way I felt violated. I felt like this girl got me drunk so she could take advantage of a younger guy.
>
> *Derek, 28*
> *Bristol, Pennsylvania*

(…and how not to)

How to Lose Your Virginity

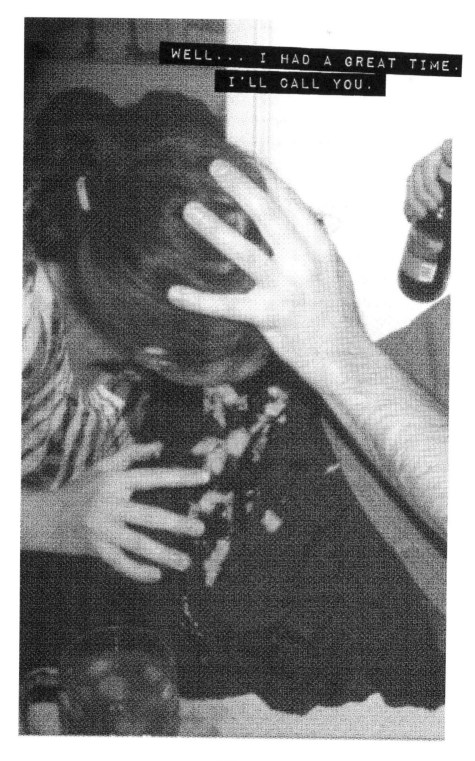

(...and how not to)

"IT WAS A TRAIN WRECK."

10

Nobody plans to have a disastrous first time, but some disasters are unavoidable. Sometimes the disaster is immediately apparent. Other times, for example with an unexpected pregnancy, reality hits weeks later. In the case of Raul's story, the discovery of disaster was delayed over a longer period, and that disaster snowballed and continued for years later.

As stated in the song "Let's Talk About Sex" by the group TLC, "Let's talk about all the good things and the bad things that may be..." Presented here are a few cautionary tales about the first time and sex in general.

THE SHERIFF'S DAUGHTER
Kenneth, 40

My parents told me nothing whatsoever about sex. Dad's an atheist, he never verbally said I love you but he finally wrote it in a card when I was 15. Kind of a sterile family, we weren't much into hugging. Thank god for my sister, Peggy. She was like, "Penis and vagina. You have a baby," and I thought, "Well I gotta avoid that. Don't want that to happen.

I loved the television show *Police Woman*. One night, I think I was 13, I had this wet dream that Angie Dickinson was on top of me with no clothes on. Then I realized penis and vagina, something comes out. I get it. That's how I fit the pieces together.

When I was 16-years-old I met a 15-year-old gal at a birthday party in Franklin, Tennessee. I liked her. And the only reason I liked her was because she liked me. I was so shy but, "Oh, someone likes me." We hang out and I turn 17, she turns 16. Then I turn 18, she turns 17. When I turned 18 her father, who was a part-time Williamson County sheriff's officer, forbade us from seeing each other any more. Her parents figured that we were doing it or we were very close. And they were right, we had just done it a few weeks before.

She had lied and told her parents that she was spending the night at a girlfriend's house. Instead we got a room at a hotel, I think it was on the corner of Lafayette or maybe Murphy Spur Rd and Spence Lane, the one behind the Huddle House. It cost $39, which back then was a good chunk of change.

We had the hymen problem. Took hours, finally we made progress with that in the morning because at one point in the evening we stopped and were exhausted from trying. In the morning we made the "break-through" and a week or two later her parents said, "We forbid you from seeing each other anymore," so we eloped. Kind of a loophole to be together, but not really the best reason to get married. The parents should have left us alone, but they forced the issue and the exact opposite of what they wanted to happen, happened.

Anyway, we got married. It was a bizarre wedding. My friend's homosexual father presided over the ceremony at a Methodist Church. Some transvestites were witnesses. She ran away from home, technically, and I secretly stashed her in a hotel, splitting my time between there and living at my mom's.

My wife's sheriff dad calls up my mom and says, "So where's Kenneth?" She says, bless her heart, "Oh, he works at the West End Cooker at West End Avenue." I ended up having to tell some customers, "I'm sorry but Willis will be taking over your table now. You can settle out with him because I have to go to jail." He showed up at the restaurant and arrested me for contributing to the delinquency of a minor. We head down to Williamson County and I made bail in 30 minutes after a good friend of mine came through with the money. That really pissed her dad off.

Yeah, we eloped and were together for two years. Didn't work out, unfortunately. Not the reason to get married but I did marry the gal I broke my virginity with.

(...and how not to)

DAD'S "FRIEND"
Russ, 27

So I was about 12, 13 years old. My father has a fruit stand in the Italian market in Philly, right where Rocky runs through in the movie. My dad says, "I know this girl." He told me to go to her house on some particular day and that she'd "take care of me."

    I saw her once. She opened the door. I went inside and it was very, very low, low-cost housing. She was older. She had tattoos. She had two kids, the whole nine yards. She was about 23, 24. She had a husband. A friend of hers was there and this friend took her two kids, who were like 2 years old and zero, to the backyard 'cause I was gonna fuck their mom.

    The mother starts blowing me. She sucked it. She sucked it, she sucked it... and I never got sucked before, but I couldn't get it going. I was laying on the floor, on the carpet, looking up at the ceiling and I'm just seeing like flies buzzing around the ceiling, mating. Finally she climbed on top of me and I'm trying to do her. I got a condom on, I'm trying to do her with the condom on. Finally I was like, "It's not gonna work. I can't cum." So she sucks it again for a little while and makes me cum orally. I spend the rest of the night showering at my grandmother's house, repeatedly, 'cause I thought I caught AIDS. I was just a child.

    I talked with my dad about it and I said, "Dad, I think I got AIDS." One of many moments in my life where my dad was like, "Maybe I made a mistake."

    I don't know if he paid her. I don't know who she was. Maybe he knew her from the market. I don't even want to think about it.

> When I sobered up in the morning I went back to that hill and I couldn't find any of my clothes or my wallet. I didn't even remember exactly where I went that night but... I just remember very vividly that we were behind that house and I lost everything, almost everything I had out on that trip. Luckily this was before 9/11 and they never questioned who I was or where I was going and I walked on the plane to get home with no ID.
>
> *Greg, 23*
> *New York, New York*

THE RIPPLE EFFECT
Raul D, 31

SHAWN WICKENS: So tell me about the first time.

RAUL D: The whole history?

SW: As much as you want to give.

RD: Think it was the summer of '89...

SW: High School?

RD: Not even. I had just graduated grammar school, eighth grade. It was some girl I dated during grammar school.
    I grew up in Jersey. And uh... very attractive girl. You know, we did our puppy love dating. According to her I was her first love. You know, that's the first time I ever got in some sort of relationship. We never did anything. We broke up, we maintained as friends 'cause we were in the same school in the same grade. Then I think it led up to the summer when we parted ways. My best friend at the time, he was much older than me and he used to give me these stories about getting laid, how it was great. I thought, "Shit. My best friend is getting laid and not me."

SW: He turned you on to drinking and stuff...

RD: Oh, he turned me on to a lot of things. We don't even talk anymore. He was my best friend, you know. I looked up to him a lot. So whatever, I was like, "Fuck. I want to get laid." So, opportunity came... I think it was actually the last day of school, maybe not summer yet.

SW: This was after you were dating?

RD: Yeah this was after, like we just kept on being friends. But I didn't get laid, I was going home and jerking off. The opportunity rose when on the last day of school, she invited me over. A bunch of us were supposed to go to her house for some sun tanning on the roof of her house. And I ended up being the only one there. So the opportunity presented itself.

SW: It was fate.

RD: Oh, I guess. And her younger brother, she had a much younger brother, he was watching TV so I was like, "Fuck it. Let me just go for it all." And we did and we got down to it and I was all eager to getting involved and getting it done and, you know, we were in the bed fooling around and I'm trying to work it. Here I am – I got an erection, I got her naked and I'm ready to go. I'm trying to find her fucking vagina. I couldn't find it for shit. So I was like, "Damn what's going on?"

(...and how not to)

In the back of my head I was thinking, you know, I hear stories that you have to break the hymen and all that stuff. So I just kept on pushing, I remember I just kept on pushing. And then I guess I finally penetrated and it just swam right in there. And it hurt me more than it hurt her. I was like in pain. And then the next thing that popped in my head was, "Wow this thing is really hot. Hot and slippery."

I did the deed. I was all... during the time I was having sex I was loving it, but in the back of my head I like couldn't wait to run back and tell my best friend that I finally got laid. So that's how that happened. That day. Finally did it and that's exactly what I did, I went to my best friend's house and told him what happened.

SW: Did you even tan at all?

RD: No we went straight into it and then once I was done I bailed right out. That's basically the first time. And the story gets a weird twist because um... she ended up, well I never saw her again. Believe it or not that last day of school was the last time I saw her.

My sophomore year, maybe third quarter of the year and she came back to school, she started going to the same high school so I was interested in where she'd been. She said she had to talk to me about a real big thing. I was like, "Where you been? I haven't seen you around." It ended up that time I lost my virginity, she ended up getting pregnant. So she... she bore my child, my first-born.

SW: So she had the baby?

RD: She had the baby. It's kind of, this is where it gets ugly. So she was ashamed and... her father was giving her problems. So her mom shipped her off back to her country. She was Dominican. She was shipped off and she had the baby and then she came back. So I was like, "Whoa I have a kid?" you know. It was like two years later. I was like 16, man. I was like, "Holy shit." At the time I was playing all these sports. I was young, starting to be a teenager. And then it hit me, "How am I gonna explain this to my family?" I knew my mom would have kicked the shit out of me. She says we have to talk about it after school, we'll meet up. So I felt obligated to meet up with her.

I ended up meeting up with her and... we talked a little bit and what happened was the baby was born with a heart defect and the baby died like maybe a couple of weeks later. And it was buried over there in that country. And she handed me a picture so I actually got to see my first-born and it was a boy.

That crushed me and it may sound fucked up, but... as much as I was scared I was kind of happy that it happened. It worked out 'cause I would have been a teenage dad. But you also can't help but feel horrible and responsible, in a way, for what happened to her afterwards 'cause she was having all these problems about the baby.

SW: Emotional problems?

RD: I know it hit her hard. She was having all these problems emotionally and with her family and then after that I rarely ever saw her again. So I had this whole secret. I never even told anybody, really, except my best friend. My mom doesn't even know to this day. I have this little chest that I keep the picture in, you know.

This story gets a real twist in it. I was in high school, I was succeeding in sports, I was gonna play ball, I was a musician also, so I had this whole thing going and it's all because I had this opportunity of what happened, you know of the baby dying, that I was able to achieve these things.

She went through a downward spiral. She got kicked out of the house, started living in the streets. It was… it really got bad for her. I would maybe run into her once every five years or something like that, and I ran into her last summer and um… here goes the other speech, she goes, I have to talk to you. And I was like, "Whatever. What could it be?" We talked and the last time I saw her, she was dancing at a strip bar. I just ended up walking in and there she was, you know. She was talking to me and then… it ended up… and I haven't seen her since this whole conversation… she said she wanted me to go with her, back to her country to make a special ceremony for the baby. And I was like, "I'll give you that." And I was like, "Why? What's going on?" And then she tells me that she was HIV-positive and she has AIDS. So… like… in that instant…

SW: It's heart-breaking.

RD: I just think of that one day that it was a pure lustful act for me to… just to satisfy not only myself but to tell my best friend what I had accomplished, but what did I really accomplish? I don't know if that little emotional damage just triggered a whole series of events for her that made things get worse. I don't know. But I have to live with that. And it sucks. So it's kind of a yin and yang thing, you know, it was great but… it was great short-term but the long-term it… not only destroyed two lives but the aftershock of it affected everyone else who was involved.

SW: It sounded like she had a pretty unsupportive family too.

RD: It was tumultuous. But… I don't know. I wasn't there. And I hate it because me being glad came at the price of the death of my first-born. And now, not only the death of my first-born but, now the death of my first-born's mother.

SW: No kids since then?

RD: Me? No. After that, no. I don't know if her condition is worse now. I haven't seen her since maybe two years ago. I'd like to say it's been tough for me but I didn't really have a tough time. I wasn't around. There was no emotional attachment. That act was done prior to my freshman year. And here I am a man, as much as I can think of myself as a man because of the situation. But I'm doing great, personally. That one little thing… it's surprising how fragile life… the smallest detail you can do to change it. How it just… you're not looking but behind the scenes there's a whole other map of the series of events that you can't control.

(...and how not to)

SHORE LEAVE
Billy, 59

This was in 1965 or '66. Something like that. Probably '66. Maybe '65. Stationed in Turkey and my second day there some guys took me to this brothel. It was like a brothel but the girls were actually prisoners, stuck there for breaking the law and made to work as like call girls. They had guards stationed at the gate and they'd let us in because we were American soldiers. I went in there and it was a terrible experience, I was very, very, very uptight about it. I felt so guilty for myself. But I'm sure the girl felt worse than I did.

WELL... I HAD A GREAT TIME. I'LL CALL YOU.
Alisa, 23

I was drinking at my friend's house, getting pretty drunk. It was the '90s and we thought we were so cool. We were all drinking 40s of Old E'. I had been partying for about a year by then. This guy I really liked, who I had a big crush on and would never even give me the time of day was there. Everybody left to go on a beer run or get pot or something.

It was just the two of us. I was wearing army pants and this big sweater. It was so cute, he stuck his head up underneath my sweater and came up through the top so his face was right in front of mine. He looked at me and he asked if I wanted to go to his house and play video games. I was 16, I was so shy, hadn't really yet developed all that much. Very, very naïve. So we went around the corner to his house and we didn't play any video games.

We fooled around. We drank some more, smoked a little bit. I tried to go down on him but I threw up all over his small penis. Then he went inside me and I asked him, "Is that it? Is there more?" It was in fact his whole penis and I felt really embarrassed. He was on top and he asked me if I wanted to do it in other positions, but I was too embarrassed so that was it. He took me back to my friend's house.

My older sister, who was 19 at the time, happened to show up there. She was a little pissed that I had done it. We took a cab home and stopped for hot dogs and had a good sister talk about the whole thing.

SEEING DOUBLE
Sandra, 24

I was in 7th grade and I was dating a guy named Norman Weller. He was a friend of a friend who lived in a different town. I hardly saw him, so our dates were phone-dates. We called each other every night, talked about shit, about having sex. "I've never had sex. Have you ever had sex?" "No."

We planned it weeks in advance. My neighbors were going out for the whole night and I was babysitting their one-year-old daughter. Norman came over and he brought his cousin with him.

The cousin must have been 16 or 17, a few years older. And Norman was obviously intimidated by his cousin. It was like the classic alpha male and beta male hierarchy thing. I remember this cousin was so sure of himself, of what he was doing, he was like, "Wait. Let me go first." I was like, "I didn't know I was going to have sex with you." But I was so young it was almost like, "OK. Whatever you want." Instead of my boyfriend, I had sex with the cousin, who I didn't even know, on my neighbors' bed while my boyfriend stood in the corner and watched.

They brought the condoms. It was so lewd, but I was scared so I went along with it. These people whose house we were in were weird; we found bullets on their night table, which made me nervous. The cousin devirginized me while my boyfriend was having a ball doing his thing. I had never even seen an erection before and here I was seeing two. There was this distinct shock at the realization that something comes out of the penis when I watched my boyfriend finish all over these weird people's bed. I wanted to have sex with him then, but he couldn't get it up again, which I thought was really funny.

I didn't want to leave any evidence so I cleaned up the mess, the bed and stuffed the paper towels in my purse and took them home. And I never actually got to have sex with that boyfriend because I hardly saw him and it just eventually ended.

> We had sex on my boyfriend's friend's living room floor. And this was after I had just thrown up on him, like ten minutes before we started fooling around. We finish and he falls asleep on the couch. I look down and it's bright red on this guy's white carpet. I sat there trying to clean this up and eventually I passed out. His friend comes downstairs the next morning and he's like, "What the hell is this? What the hell is this red stain on my carpet?" We told him I was drinking vodka with Kool-Aid."
>
> *Yolanda, 28*
> *Ann Arbor, Michigan*

(...and how not to)

I CAN'T BELIEVE I'M TELLING THIS
Bryce, 40

I was 16 or 17. My upstairs neighbors were two brothers who were about four years older than me. They were both gorgeous guys and I had a crush on both of them and they knew it. They were both bisexual so they were dating women and men. One day Craig, the older brother, took me down to the basement and I gave my first blowjob. He shot a load in my mouth so I'm guessing I did OK.

Then this other time, his brother Stan asked me if I'd ever been fucked before. I told him no and he asked, "Would you like to try it?" Not one of my best experiences. I nearly bled to death but I survived it after a lot of Preparation H and ice cubes up my butthole.

One of the them is married with two beautiful kids now, but we're all still very close.

> I used to have just fleeting thoughts about sex in my brain but after that moment I couldn't stop thinking about having sex. Whether it's sleeping, waking moments of my life I always have girls on the brain. Before that first time I actually had plans and thoughts of doing things and stuff. Sex: worst mistake I ever made.
>
> *Peter, 33*
> *Westlake, Ohio*

BEDSIDE MANNER
Shannon, 38

I was 13 when I got my period and my mom was of the school of thought that once you get your period, you need to get a checkup from the gynecologist to make sure everything is OK. So I went to the gynecologist over at Women and Infants Hospital. He goes to look at me and because I was tiny, in those days they used those awful silver clamps, he jams the clamps in there... *BAM*, that's it. Blood everywhere. I cried. I screamed. He apologized but that didn't change the fact I was totally robbed of my virginity.

I told my mom there was blood but my mom was a very strict, Irish mom. Like you wouldn't ever mention sex to her, never mind, you know, "Hey, the doctor just took care of me, thank you very much." But that was it and I was frightened to ever go back there. But maybe it was a good thing because maybe the first guy I slept with wasn't worth losing a cherry over.

RIPPED INTO ADULTHOOD
Xander A., 32

XANDER A: I'm from Texas in this small town called Alvin outside of Houston. I was like a New Wave kid in the '80s and my sister... my sister was two years younger than me so wanting to be like her big brother she was a New Waver, too.

So she had her little friends, I won't lie... I'm not proud of it, but I would listen to hear which one of her friends was going to spend the night because then after my sister would fall asleep they would sneak out and come to my room. Now my room wasn't in the house. We lived in a big wooden house and there was a storm shelter in the backyard. So I moved down there to start doing drugs and do everything they talk about in the book *Fear and Loathing in Las Vegas*... so my sister's friends would sneak out and come downstairs well... her friend Lana came down.

SHAWN WICKENS: Your sister didn't find out about it?

XA: She knew that her friends would come down but she didn't say anything, you know. But it was just kind of known. So I would always keep an ear out, "Oh. Mary is staying the night? Oh, hell yeah." Friends would ask me, "You going out Friday?" "Hell no." So... Lana came over one night and we made out and... it wasn't like today where you can just turn on the TV and know how to do anything. I didn't have HBO. I wasn't an idiot but everything I had learned was from Frederick's of Hollywood catalogs.

Anyways... I had an 8-track player... the shed in the backyard was like a clubhouse room. So I found an 8-track player and, no lie, we were talking and laughing and listening to *The Muppet Movie* soundtrack, which is a fantastic soundtrack. I had no idea that one day I would lose my virginity to this soundtrack. But, this turns into a kind of tragic, painful situation for me. I knew that it hurt girls, losing their virginity. So, you know we... Muppets are going on and it started out with, "Why are there so many songs about rainbows?" So that was the sexy song. Brother now I'm playing the, "Moving right along... foot loose and fancy free." That's when I started getting it on, bro.

So anyways we are making out and we attempt and... and I'm looking for it and I had practiced so well with my erections since I was 12. If you would have left a wallet out I would have had sex with it but I think I speak on behalf of all the boys at 12 with their Fredericks of Hollywood.

We're going and I remember it hurting really bad and I thought, "But I thought this was supposed to hurt only the girls." And she goes, "What are you talking about?" No I didn't say that out loud. But, so anyways it hurts, and we kind of finished and I'd never actually been inside someone. And so anyways so... I went to pee and I remember it hurting, passionately. This is a true story, I'm not making any of this up. So I'm peeing and it hurts so bad. I looked down and I had caused a small tear in the head of my penis, no lie.

SW: What?!

(...and how not to)

XA: No lie. And it gets worse... so now I'm torn, and it hurts. Any other time when I cut myself, not that I made a habit at 15 of doing this but when I cut myself I would go to mom. Not going to mom with this, you know because, "Serves you right. You were having sex... sin! Sin."

SW: Were you from a religious family?

XA: Oh, my mother is a Pentecostal minister, bro. But anyways... so I've torn the head of my penis and what do I think to do? This is not a fucking lie. I grabbed a bottle of alcohol... rubbing alcohol. No lie. I'm 15... I am a dumb kid. And this is a 1980s 15-year-old. Not a year 2000 15-year-old, which is the equivalent of a 27-year-old. So there is still some innocence in me. Anyways so, it's like four in the morning 'cause my moves took forever.

SW: This was on a school night?

XA: Yeah, this is on a school night.

SW: Was she there assisting you at this point?

XA: Oh no, no, no, no, no... no she was, sorry... I had gone into the house. She was still outside.

SW: Did she know about any of the tragedy that...

XA: No, I just told her I went to pee and the reason I... 'cause normally I would have just gone in the bushes, it's Texas. So I'm peeing, and I get the bottle of alcohol... and it's like four or five in the morning and I pour some on and I swear to God, bro, I saw into the future! It fucked me up and I let out a yell like, "Arghhhhhhhhh God! Oh nooooo-ahhh..." 'cause I mean, dude, you know head of a penis is a sensitive part. Tear, alcohol. I didn't know, you know. I wasn't going to put a Band-Aid on it. Nothing stupid like that... no, I did something smart like put alcohol on it. Severe pain. And so to end my virginity story... I got the virginity out of the way and the next day dropped acid at school for the first time, so did the acid and the virginity all in one day. That's the end of my story. Oh, and I healed nicely.

SW: Were you compelled to try acid because you were in pain?

XA: I knew I was going to try acid the day before, I didn't know I was going to lose my virginity that night because I didn't know my sister was going to have Lana spend the night. Life gives you lemons, bro, you tear the head of your dick.

SW: How was it, on the side or right on top? Like it made the hole bigger?

XA: No, no, no, no. Right on top. Oh that would've been terrible... now you're talking crazy shit. Can you imagine? Oh God I don't want to imagine.

SCHOOL'S OUT FOR SUMMER
Dimitri, 28

First of all, I'm gay. I am now anyway. But when I was 13 I was visiting relatives out in Long Island; out in Hicksville, Long Island, of all places. I was up there one summer staying with my cousin Zack who was this really hot Italian boy my age and I so had a crush on him. I justified my crush because he's not my first cousin, so I could probably do him, but he's not gay. Zack had a crush on this girl named Tiffany Berkley.

Tiffany had an older sister Adriane. Tiffany was a year older than us and Adriane was 16. It was the first time I met her. We went over to Zack's middle school and outside of all those old public school buildings there's those stairs, those cement stairs that lead down to a pit and the doors for the boiler room. That's where we went, down in that pit. Zack's hooking up with Tiffany and I'm stuck with this Adriane girl, the sister, who I was totally NOT into. She was actually a cute, beautiful girl but I'm a homosexual. I knew it then, whatever, I know it now.

The only thing that made me horny was the fact that 12 feet away from me, Zack was fooling around with Tiffany. Hot. He's still unmarried so there's hope. Anyway, Adriane and I were hooking up and she's reaching in and then she pulls down my pants and all this nonsense. So she's ready to go, she's ready to go and we're stripping and I think, "Aw, shit."

We all have sex. I'm in her and she's like, "Ehhh, I can't feel a thing." The whole thing was gross. The whole vagina thing was just nasty to me. That sealed the deal for my homosexuality because my first memory of sex was going down into this cold cement pit leading into a boiler room. I was against the steps with this girl on top of me, her hands on the metal railings. My back was all scraped and scratched up, and she was just going to town on me. It was horrendous.

Of course Zack thought it was the hottest thing ever that I scored and he scored too. I can remember the coldness of the metal and not wanting to do it. *Ugh*, I'm really happy that I'm homosexual.

There was a laundry chute in the bathroom so I snuck into the bathroom and climbed down through the laundry chute. My girlfriend walked down through the kitchen, met me in the basement and let me out of the house. I scratched my back up pretty severely, but managed to keep the escape pretty quiet.

Luke, 25
Nashville, Tennessee

(...and how not to)

UNREQUITED SEX
Stacy, 21

He was my first real, real boyfriend. Six months into the relationship I thought I loved the kid. We wound up doing it on my bed at 5 o'clock in the morning. My mom was right next door. It fucking sucked. In the meantime I was trying to make it better so I said, "I love you," and he never said it back. I was stupid and 16. There are times when a guy wants to reciprocate and pleasure the girl and this was definitely the kind of first experience where he was just trying to get off. I thought I loved him and he didn't love me and that hurt real bad.

The next day I had a grotesque bathroom experience at an all-day concert and spent a lot of time doubled over in an outhouse – wasn't used to the whole cherry-breaking.

> It was in a car, a Mustang, the back seat. I got pregnant but it's gone. It... ceased to exist. I was 15.
>
> *Karen, 23*
> *Medina, Ohio*

DOWNHILL
Lacey, 22

I was 17 and used to ski competitively – slalom, GS, super-8, whatever, and I met this guy at a ski race. He was in a competitive class above me and we were on the top of some mountain when he turned his head my way so I thought, "All right, sweet. I got some college guy's attention."

He invited me to a party back at his condo and I went with a couple of my younger girlfriends and we drank... a bunch. It was probably like my first or second time getting drunk. He took me up to the attic where everyone was laying in their respective make out piles. I was really fucked up and thought I was so cool because I had a college guy. Then it became like the situation at the beginning of *Kids* with Tully saying to that girl, "Yeah, you're doing great. You're doing great. Keep on going. We're almost there." And I was saying, "No. It hurts. Stop." 'Cause seriously, and not to be vulgar, but it was a huge penis. I'm 22 now and I've seen other penises since then and I still consider his to be huge.

So it sucked, it was a terrible experience and later on at the party someone told me the guy was still dating his 25-year-old girlfriend. It was awful. I was traumatized. I didn't have sex for like two more years after that because I just hated it. And on top of all that, he told his friends that I was a prude and that I wouldn't even have sex with him, which I did. I did have sex with him, it felt horrible, and he lied about it.

ALL I WANTED WAS FOR SOMEONE TO BE THERE WHEN I NEEDED
Deborah O, 21

DEBORAH O: I got kicked out; my parents are divorced and I got kicked out of my mom's house and I moved in with my dad. And then a month later he started going through a divorce from his second wife.

SHAWN WICKENS: Was this in the same town?

DO: Yes. It was in the same town, everything. Well, my brother was kicked out earlier so pretty much I was cut off from everyone in my family. My dad was going insane and I wasn't on speaking terms with my mom and my brother was nowhere to be found. And my dad wouldn't let me speak with my stepmom. So I didn't have anybody. Plus I switched high schools all at the same time and... I was 16. I started hanging out with... not a bad crowd, I was just used to being a straight-A student and so I got into drugs and alcohol and skipping school and all that stuff when I met this guy named Orlando Ortiz. He was Dominican. I was young, I was 16, I was just of age, you know, legally I would say. And I really, really liked him. I thought he was beautiful.

SW: Can you remember the day you two met?

DO: Yeah, I do remember. We were at a party and I knew that he really liked me, but just initially, from the looks, from the natural vibe, but I wasn't that interested. It was more when I got to know him and the little things like the slight accent, when he would drink you could hear it a little bit more and... I liked the fact that he treated me like I was too young to be sexual. Like in some way it gave me an advantage that everyone thought I was naïve. I hung out with him and our whole group of friends every single night 'til about 4 o'clock in the morning.

SW: You were still at your dad's at this point?

DO: Yeah. But my dad, he stayed out really late. He was really messed up emotionally, too. So finally, the fact that I had this tremendous crush on him just came out but he had feelings for one of my older friends... but she didn't like him.

SW: He shared this with you?

DO: Yeah... I mean, it was obvious. And I was so young too, and naïve... so he called me one night when he was really drunk and asked me to come pick him up to give him a ride... *ugh*, this is such an awful story. I really, really liked him and I picked him up and gave him a ride and then we decided to go to the beach. We were on the sand, near the ocean and we started making out and then we went to the lifeguard post and had sex on the lifeguard post and then went back to the car.

SW: Him sort of sitting down and you on top of him, I guess...

DO: No, no, no. Well it ended up we were standing and then it was just too painful so I had lay down and then he was on top.

(...and how not to)

SW: Was it just a chair or was it a large...

DO: No, it was the lifeguard post like the big structures they have on the beach. It was pitch dark, a little bit windy and the sand was uncomfortable and all that kind of stuff but... so we walked back to the car and that's when I realized how drunk he actually was. And then when we got back in the car, I remember it was a CD we listened to... Ginuwine, do you know which one I'm talking about, anyways it's the ridiculous album with the song "So Anxious" on it*. So we made out for that whole album.

I dropped him off at his house and we made out for like a good 40 minutes. I remember the whole day afterwards wondering if he was going to call and he never did and he didn't call for a whole week. And then I saw him at one of the gatherings.

SW: At a house party?

DO: No, it was actually outside, it was a big keg party or something like that. He saw me and said, "Oh, hi," and he gave me a kiss on the cheek and then he went on to go flirt with other girls. Highly painful. And then when I talked to him about it later I said, "What's going on?" He goes, "What? I'm always nice to you. I always give you a kiss on the cheek." And I said, "Well, Orlando, you always give everybody a kiss on the cheek." And all he could do was laugh 'cause he was embarrassed because it was almost like I called him out and he had guilt about it... but not enough pride or not enough integrity as a man to even talk about it. But at the same time I knew that he wasn't mature enough to take responsibility for the fact that he was not sober and I was sober and I willingly, you know, gave my virginity away.

His friend gave me a call and asked me if I was a virgin anymore and I said, "No why?" And he goes, I was just wondering. I said, "Why would you ask me that?' And he goes, "I was just wondering." 'Cause they all knew that I was a virgin and then... so...

SW: Maybe he didn't remember it happening?

DO: No, I think Orlando was bragging about it. And that upset me. I realized that he may have been older than me but he was less mature and I just felt... 1) hurt, taken advantage of and 2) really, really naïve all at the same time and it changed my view on men and on relationships from then on.

SW: And plus your parents were divorced and your dad was remarried and he was getting divorced. Were you more hopeful about relationships in general before then?

DO: No. My stepmom was cheating on my father for like the whole ten years they were together. I just felt like there was betrayal everywhere I went. It wasn't that I wanted to have sex with him, I just wanted some sort of relationship. You know, some sort of love and then when I realized that that's not what sex was... it... really messed me up. I got depressed to the point that it affected my body because I no longer wanted anyone to find me attractive. So, looking back on it now I subconsciously started gaining weight and I stopped shaving my legs just because I didn't want to go through the same experience.

SW: Did he see you during this self-imposed unattractive phase?

DO: I removed myself from the crowd. I went back to my old high school... my father and I started going to therapy... I didn't speak with my stepmom anymore but my mom and I got in a relationship again and, well... on top of all that stuff happening I thought I had cancer.

SW: How did you think you had cancer?

DO: This was awful. I was under so much stress from my mom's house. I was a really good kid, I didn't deserve to get kicked out. I think she was menopausal and I was the typical emotional teenager, you know, anyway I was feeling so emotionally abused that I was bleeding rectally from the stress.

SW: I would think cancer too then.

DO: Yeah, yeah, yeah. Well, I had to get a colonoscopy... my like GI guy, my specialist told me that I needed a colonoscopy 'cause he thought that I had cancer or something like that. And it ended up it was just stress. But I had to do all the medical appointments and everything by myself. I had emotional support. I had all the financial support I could want but all of it means shit... you know?

SW: Well there was a silver lining. You got your dad into therapy.

DO: Yeah. I was always the advocate to wait until marriage and then it was just ironic that once my dad and my stepmom who I had considered a perfect marriage, split up, that's when I lost my virginity. Now I don't believe in the institution of marriage whatsoever. My dad got remarried and now he has a baby. His new wife is manic-bipolar. I just have no fucking faith and it's awful and I think it's a product of how I was raised.

* 100% Ginuwine

A LOT OF MONEY BACK THEN
Bob, 42

Many moons ago I was 16, my girlfriend was 15, and we both decided to break our virginities together.

Maybe I had the condom on for too long, it was on the whole time during foreplay. But when I pulled it out the rubber was broken. She didn't have a period for a while, then we went and got a test. Knocked her up – had to pay for an abortion. That cost $135 at the time. Paid for it with money I made working as a cart boy at Target.

We were both too young. I regret it, though of course by now I could be a grandpa, were my child to have made the same mistake.

Other than that it was fun.

(...and how not to)

THE AFTERMATH
Ed, 45

Junior year some of my friends and I struck up a friendship with our English teacher. She was fairly new; I think it was her first teaching experience right after college. She was a pretty cool teacher. She was newly divorced from her childhood sweetheart who was a heck of a high school athlete in his own right, and she was living in a trailer out in Lincoln. Various weekends she would invite us out to her trailer and we would drink and party with her and her new boyfriend.

This one night... during our Christmas vacation, I distinctly remember it was the Sunday night before we were to go back to school. I get home from pumping gas out on I-80 and my dad said there was a phone call for me but they didn't leave a message. The phone rang again and it was a couple of my friends saying they were at our teacher's trailer and they wanted me to stop over.

By the time I got there she was pretty liquored up. My friends were liquored up too but not as bad as she was. One thing led to another and we were in the hallway shooting beers, spraying each other. A few of the guys got their shirts wet and took them off and she started making out with us, going from guy to guy. Pretty soon her and one of my buddies went into her bedroom. They were in there quite a while and so we pop the door open and we could see the old white ass bouncing up and down. After he was done he came flying out and another buddy went in there. Then I was third, same thing. Went in there and it was my first time and all. As I'm going at it she's yelling, "Nick! Nick!" the name of the first guy. After I was done the fourth guy went in. Evidently she sobered up because she cut him off.

The bad thing about it was the next day we go back to school expecting to face her but she's not there. She didn't show up until three days later and pretty bruised up. Turns out her boyfriend came back that night after we left, figured out what happened and beat the crap out of her.

Being from a small town and stuff, you know, loose lips go flying and people hear about stuff. To this day, here I am in my 40s and whenever I go back to Nebraska I still get people coming up to me and asking me if that's true.

Running home I jumped this three-bar wooden fence and as I stepped on the top plank it snapped, sending me down into the mud. Everything was against me after that horrible event, even nature.

Mack, 27
Sheffield, England

YOU FUCKED CATHY CAPPIZIOTTI.
Tom, 34

I had been distressed for the entire summer after I graduated high school because I wanted to get laid before I turned 18 and I was to turn 18 that November during my first semester in college. I figured there was no way I was going to get to college and in just two or three short months convince any of this new pool of women to sleep with me, so I needed to get laid before college.

I had a friend who tried to help me out that summer setting me up with various girls, all this nonsense. Nothing worked. He even tried to convince his own girlfriend to sleep with me. That poor girl had to say she was on her period for like three months straight. College starts, the 18th birthday comes and goes in early November, I go home for Thanksgiving break and I'm all down in the mouth about my big failure; I'm 18 and still a virgin.

I'm hanging out with some friends who were in the class behind me and there was one girl there: Cathy Cappiziotti. For my group of friends, Cathy had been the object of our abuse for the last six months of my senior year of high school 'cause she had gotten this huge crush on a friend of mine. She sent him a letter saying how she was all crazy about him and included the lyric to The Eagles' song "Desperado," "Come down from your fences," you know, "...let down your defenses." Like she was really trying to get to this guy by saying you're so closed up but I know there's a warm heart in there somewhere. And for this very earnest gesture she of course earned all this abuse from me and my friends, this totally callous group of asshole guys.

And so we were sitting around at this party, a bunch of nerdy guys and her. All the guys were bitching about how we couldn't get any women. She was sashaying around the room talking about, "Well I have sex all the time. It's great. I feel sorry for you." And we were just like, "Fuuuck you." Everyone started heaping abuse on her but it was all pretty weak because what could we say? For all the shit we were talking, she was getting it and we weren't.

I just got disgusted with the whole affair and I went and I sat in the next room. Cathy came and sat down next to me. I had been so condescending and awful to this girl for so long that what happened next was completely beyond my grasp of psychology at the time. I don't even understand it now but she asks me, "You're lonely, aren't you?" And in a moment of drunkenness I said, "Yeah... I'm fucking lonely and I'm sick of this." And she said, "Well, why don't we?" I told myself, "Well I'm not gonna fuck her. She's got great tits but she's a little heavy for my taste," 'cause like I'm such a fucking find. I'm this skinny guy, fucking big wimp and nerd and so I said, "Maybe I'll play with your breasts." I was such a callous asshole.

Of course I do end up fucking her. It happened pretty suddenly and the other guys are banging on the door like, "What the fuck is going on in there?" And of course I didn't have a condom but she said, "I'm on the pill. Don't worry about it." I'm drunk, I'm 18, I'm like, "OK."

I was like so wigged out about AIDS, this was 1989 and at that time we were brought up to believe everyone was going to die of AIDS within five years. So I walk out stark naked and go to the bathroom to wash my dick off in the sink. "Gotta get it off. Gotta get the shame off." Like I was Lady Macbeth, incarnadining the sink with blood.

(...and how not to)

I walk back in there, and I'm 18, of course I'm ready to go again in spite of my own fears. So I fuck her again and when I come out the guys had put all these kitchen products outside the door, like Saran Wrap and Ziploc bags and tinfoil. We had this friend named Chris who told us this story about some girl who wouldn't let him fuck her because he didn't have a condom, so he was like, "I used a plastic bag man, it worked perfect." In honor of Chris they threw all that stuff out there as a joke.

Obviously I had totally caved to this girl. I got dressed and I came out all pumped up. Everyone was like, "Way to go. Got the monkey off your back," except for my best friend who was all about principle and sticking to your guns and stuff. We left her there and we went out walking around the neighborhood trying to find beer somewhere. I said to him "Man I can't believe I just fucked Cathy Cappiziotti." This was like my best friend but we were always competitive with one another. Now I was sort of one up on him a little bit, but he wasn't congratulating me or anything. All he said was, "I'll have four words for you in the morning." And the next morning I woke up out of my stupor and he's standing over me and he says, "You – fucked – Cathy – Cappiziotti." That's all he would say to me.

That next morning I regretted it, but in a way it was just like this perfect drunken stupid thing. I was supposed to be this big intellectual whatever and she was just like some average girl, but all that bullshit you connect with of finding the right girl, that magical connection, that doesn't mean anything. Looking back now, if I saw her today I'd say "thank you".

A DAY OF INFAMY
Ryan, 23

It was 9/11, the 9/11. I was a freshman at Waldorf College in Forrest City, Iowa. There was this girl I really had a crush on and she kept crying because she had family in New York.

We were both theater students. She called me up because she was far from home and she needed a friend. I went over there and I was like, "Yeah, it's really fucked up." This is really awful but I said to her, "I don't want to die a virgin." But come on, I thought the whole world was coming to an end. So we fucked in her bunk bed with her roommate asleep right there on the top bunk. She was hot and one of the most sought-after girls in the school, but she was taken. She had a boyfriend of four years and they broke up after he found out.

I feel real bad that I used other people's tragedy to get me laid, but I'm very thankful for it. Like in a way it's wrong to thank the terrorists for a bad thing that happened but it got me laid. And now I'm a firefighter so that's pretty fucked up too.

How to Lose Your Virginity

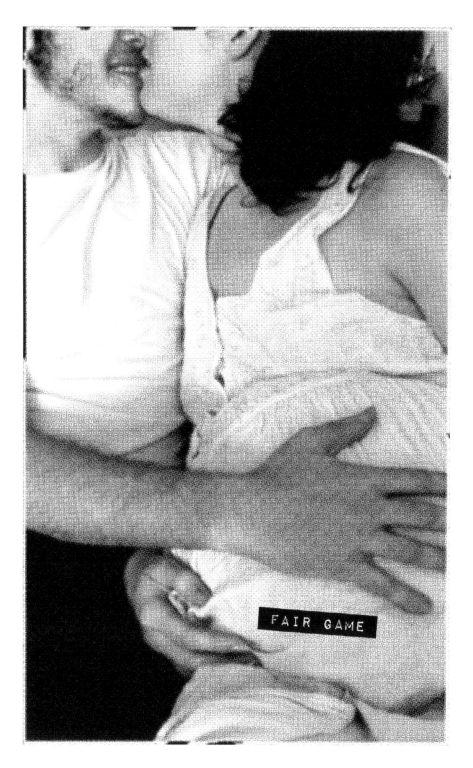

(...and how not to)

"MEN CAN BE SUCH PIGS."

11

There is probably not a woman out there (or man for that matter) who has at some point held pretty low opinions of the "stronger" sex. Guys can be creeps. Some are even proud of it.

NOM DE PLUME
Phoebe, 21

I'm from Austin but moved to Minnesota for nine years then moved to Carson City, Nevada, to live with my grandparents for six years, where it happened. I had a perm and really pasty white skin. I was a freshman in high school and I had never known popularity but when I entered high school life I found out that this senior boy thought that I was cute. I hung out with all of his friends and we started dating.

It wasn't until later that I found out the senior guys had a top ten list of the "hottest" freshman girls. It was a deflowering list and I was number two behind two girls Jen and Haley, tied at number one. The boys were too indecisive, I guess, to settle on just ten.

So this guy came up to me after school one day and I had no idea who he was. I wasn't really concerning myself with any boys, and I was a good girl. He comes up to me and he goes, "Hi, my name's Luther," like nice to meet you kind of nonchalant. He gives me his number and we hang out a few times.

Luther comes over to my house and, mind you, I had never even seen a penis in my life except for either maybe my dad's or my grandpa's. We were watching *American History X* in my bedroom. My grandparents were out at choir rehearsal for our church.

We're doing the whole make out thing and he starts trying things, which I thought, "OK, I'll go along with it." I was 14, almost 15 and when you're that age you don't know too much about grooming, which leads to an embarrassing part of the story later on. But we're there watching *American History X* and the last scene I remember was Edward Norton "curbing" some guy.

We're doing the whole rubbing on the clothes thing and he goes, "My dick is chafing, let's take our clothes off." Somehow I end up with my clothes off but he keeps all his clothes on. I'm naked, he's fully dressed.

One of my girlfriends was over at the same time but she didn't like the guy so she was in the other room using the Internet. He got me naked so he's like, "Let's try it." Of course I freak out so I tell him I have to use the bathroom and I put on a t-shirt and leave the room to go ask my girlfriend, "What should I do? What should I do?" Little did I know she was a whore, she had been doing this for God knows how long, since she was like 12. She told me, "Yeah, do it. Go for it." I go back in there and we get back to the fondling phase and he says, "All right I'm going to do it now." I tell him, "If it hurts you have to stop and I don't want you to do it anymore."

Of course he's not gentle in any way. He was literally with all his weight on me, shoving it right in. I start bawling. I'm screaming, "What are you doing?!" I'm freaking out and I look over at the TV and I can see Edward Norton getting raped in the ass.

And this is supposed to be one of the most romantic moments of my lifetime? I'm crying and I'm covering my face and he has the audacity to say, "Shut up. It'll be over soon." And it was. He finishes after a couple minutes and gets up to leave 'cause he was going to a party that night. I couldn't walk. He tries to be nice to me and gives me a piggyback ride down the stairs and I'm still, not to be gross, but I was still bleeding. Then he gives me a high five, right? Like we were football players. "Yeah, high five!"

(...and how not to)

The next day I go to school and I'm hiding from him, literally hiding behind lockers and moving friends in front of me and he didn't even care. He's not trying to talk to me either. Two days later we go to his friend's house and everyone came up to me at the party and said things like, "I heard you had sex with Luther." I was like, "How does everyone know?"

I found out that he got a hundred bucks and not only that, but everyone knew that it had happened. I had told only two of my girlfriends. He told everybody. Later that week he broke up with me and of course started dating one of my friends.

Not only that but he told everyone physical details about me and about how I, at 14, didn't know about grooming. For the next two years in high school everybody called me "Bushykins" or "Cry Baby." And his friends would constantly make sexual innuendos towards me. In my yearbook somebody wrote, "Let's *meat* behind the gym lockers," spelled M-E-A-T.

And I was the first one on the top ten list to give it up. But throughout the whole year, one would go then two would go and then four and then finally all of the top 10 were totally deflowered. But the guy who won the bet, ultimately, was a guy who screwed a girl and then screwed her mother. They had a pool going and I don't know if it's like poker or what, but the guy ended up winning a pair of Nike Air Jordans and like 500 bucks.

It was kind of an ordeal and I don't even live there anymore but to this day people know about it, still call me things. I didn't have a bad reputation beforehand but after that I got a horrible reputation so it really killed me. I ended up drinking religiously, dropping out of high school junior year and getting my GED.

That guy Luther is a dirty dog and now I think he's working at a gas station even though he's got a rich family and he's just a huge loser now and probably still living in Carson City. He's just an idiot. He was 18 and I was 14, and it was so illegal for him to do. Nowadays I just thank God that my mentality level is so much higher now and I got past it and know that I had to live through that one experience to just be like, "Fuck it. One day I'll be happy."

ONE MAN'S HAPPY MEMORY IS ANOTHER WOMAN'S REGRET
Andrew, 45

I was 15 and this friend of mine was banging this chick. One day he asked, "Hey, ever had sex?" I'm like, "No." He says, "Well I'll let you screw this girl I'm screwing." Stella was her name; we all went to school together. We went down to her place, he went in and did it, they came back out and he said Stella wants to do it. She went, "What?" But he talked her into it. So I went in her house and she done me to. Didn't kiss or nothing, we just done it. Then we had to get out of there before her parents got home 'cause she was like 13. Real sweet.

A PRICK IN SHEEP'S CLOTHING
Carol, 19

There was this guy named Jack and I had gone on a couple of dates with him. He seemed interesting. Later I found out he was a total jerk and he was just trying to get in my pants.

I guess I sort of felt pressured into it and before it happened he smoked three joints through his nostrils. He thought he was so cool that he could do that. I didn't want to do it, but he was pressuring me. We went into the bedroom and when I told him that it started to hurt, he completely didn't care. Afterwards I distinctly remember saying, "Was that it?" He said, "What? Do you expect me to cuddle or something?" and he just walked out.

After we finished the first time I felt so low about myself that he was able to get me back into the bedroom and we actually did it again, sort of like to see if it was different, if it was really worth it. It was like self-assurance but it wasn't any better.

He took me home and I just lay in bed thinking, "Oh my god, I can't believe I lost my virginity to such a prick." I couldn't believe it because he seemed like a nice guy and he went to a real good school. In the end he just really wasn't worth it. He kept calling me afterwards, but I never returned his phone calls and I've never talked to him since that day.

I spoke with my mom, sort of cried to her about it and she was very supportive. But I was upset when I found out my dad knew because I was sort of like a daddy's little girly-girl. Mom reassured me by saying, "Has your father treated you any different since he found out?" She was right, he hadn't. What he really cared about was that I was safe and OK. Since then my relationship with my mom has grown and I can talk to her about that kind of stuff even more now.

> This guy I knew, Jeremy, broke up with his girlfriend who was like the biggest slut in town because he found out she went "skiing," if you can visualize a girl doing that motion. And by skiing I mean Janelle jerked off two guys at the same time. I moved in and started hanging out with her.
>
> *Kevin, 26*
> *Seacrest Beach, New Jersey*

(...and how not to)

FAIR GAME
Roland, 31

It was with a girl in the very far suburbs and the further you get out of St. Louis, Missouri, the more trailers and farms you get. And I'm with a girl from way, way outside of St. Louis – farm and trailer park country. Her name was Caroline Arkey and I wouldn't mind finding her again and believe me, I've been looking.

We watched *Scream 2* and we're making out and the girl says to me, "Do you want to have sex?" I said, "No... I don't know." She's like, "Well I have to tell you something." "Well what is it honey?" "I have to tell you, I'm already pregnant." That was what convinced me because I couldn't get this girl more pregnant. She's already gonna have somebody else's kid. It's a free go!

She was about two months along, I guess. Barely showing but enough so that her breasts had swelled so nicely. We had sex and about 12 minutes later I packed up to leave.

So the point is, first time, lost my virginity to a pregnant girl when I was 17. Wonderful experience, she was 15, her kid now is maybe 10. Didn't use a condom. She was already pregnant, right? So what's the worst that could happen? Little did I know like about STDs. But I've given blood since then and they never called. They never called so I'm good, right?

BREAKING AND ENTERING
Yosef, 30

I met this girl at my 15th birthday party I was having at a friend's place. I was about to take her home but when you're 15 and you live with your parents and four brothers you can't just take a girl home for sex. I decided to take her to my school in Tel Aviv, Israel. I told her that my father was the sports teacher and that I had keys for the gym. Had her wait by the front door and I snuck around the back, hopped a few fences, broke a window, then opened the front door for her from the inside.

That's where I had my first sex, in the gym, in the middle of the night on those real big high jump mats – the huge ones you had to climb up to get on. I didn't know a whole lot about sex but it was fun. It was comfortable to have sex sunk deep down in that huge mattress.

That girl, I never called her and I feel bad about it now, but I just left her there in the school. She was from a different state so I don't know if she knew how to get home. I didn't even care. I just left her. Then when I got home I thought, "Geez, what about that girl?" Since then I've learned to take better care of girls.

The next morning I told all my friends like, "Yeah, I got laid on my 15th birthday in the fucking school with a fucking hot girl." They didn't believe me so I showed them the broken window.

MY DRUG BUDDY
Chip, 22

I met this girl from the neighborhood. We always got high together behind my shed. I just thought we were weed smoking buddies. I had no clue this chick liked me. I'm walking her home one night in the rain and I was like, "I'll walk you half way," such was our routine. We get to the halfway point and she's like, "I got to tell you something." "What's up? You want to smoke again?" She's like, "I like you. I want to date you." She wasn't that good looking so I ain't fuckin' dating her.

She just starts kissing me. She kind of like bum-rushed me. I think she liked me a lot because she was pretty aggressive. And it felt kind of good when she kissed me. I wasn't like blown away by it, but holy shit, I pretty much got a fucking boner from just kissing her. So I figured, "I got a boner, I might as well screw her."

We're kissing in the rain and shit. There were these woods in our neighborhood, right down the street from our halfway point. We go by the woods, and I don't know, I think she had a condom; she had to have. Maybe she planned it; I never asked. But what I do know is that we ended up fucking in the woods for two minutes. I fucking two-pump chumped her. That was about it. I had a good time so I walked her all the way home that night.

We fucked for awhile and then she wanted the relationship but I told her, "Look. I'm not doing it. I don't want to date you but we can have sex and get high behind my shed."

SECRET HANDSHAKES
Ray, 26

I dated this girl for three months which, to this day I think is still my record. Veronica and I got close but she would never sleep with me. All my friends were getting laid. Finally I just got tired of it. I called up this other girl who Veronica went to school with, a known slut, and asked her out to a movie.

I pick her up, we're driving to the theater and she asks, "Why'd you call me?" You know so, I tried my best line, "Because I really like you." And she's like, "Yeah, bullshit. Do you still want to go to this movie?" I said, "Well what are some other options?" She said, "I don't know. What else is there to do?" So I took her over to my buddy Kurt's place.

Kurt had this playhouse we'd play in as kids. But it was a big playhouse. It had bunk beds and all that B.S. Three of my buddies lost their virginity there. We called it the "Stabbin' Cabin". It had no lights so all of us had Indiglo watches to work the combination lock on the outside door. And it was all coordinated, you get inside and the lights wouldn't work so you had to sleep together. There was a stash of condoms and when you were done you'd just throw them in the fireplace. Every Saturday morning we'd get together and burn up the used ones.

This all got back to my ex-girlfriend, it being with a girl she knew, so she showed up at my house in tears, absolute tears but I was away at basketball camp. My old man had a talk with me when I got back. But yeah, that was the Stabbin' Cabin.

(...and how not to)

HIJACKED
Dave, 23

It's the start of my first year at college and I'm anticipating meeting a chick at some keg party or somewhere, who will take my virginity. That's how I thought it would go down but it didn't quite happen that way.

A couple seniors on my hockey team came over to my room and said, "Hey you want to go and blow lines all night?" I said, "Yeah. I'll blow lines with you guys." I figure, "Hell, why not," so I go and blow lines with them. They say cocaine is supposed to limit your sex drive but it didn't stand in my way that night.

After a ton of partying it's 6:30 in the morning and we're riding around in this one guy's Ford Explorer. We're going crazy, going stupid and we see this girl walking back from some apartment. So we're like, "Yo. What's up? Want to get into our car?" She gets in. I figure we're gonna go get breakfast.

These guys start saying shit like, "We're gonna take you out to the woods and rape the shit out of you. We're gonna fucking tie you to a tree." She understandably gets freaked out. I try calming her down, telling her that they're just joking. Meanwhile we turn off the street down some farm road. The whole time the driver is going on and on about how they're going to chop off her legs and all this weird shit. We were all coked up.

She's like, "What the fuck's going on?" I say, "Don't worry, honey. Everything's gonna be OK. These guys aren't that bad." Meanwhile she's getting more and more frightened and they turn off into a farm.

They slam on the brakes, corn stalks seven to eight feet tall on either side of us. She jumps out balling her eyes out. I go chasing after her, I'm like, "Listen. They're lying. It's no big deal." Somehow I get her back into the car. We go to the breakfast place. It's all over with, but she's still shaken up.

After breakfast, she and I went back to my dorm room. She's still whacked out, asking me, "What were those guys thinking? I was so afraid for my life." I massaged her shoulders to calm her down. Howard Stern came on the radio, he had a stripper on or something funny like that. She loosens up, starts laughing a little bit. We got to talking and then things happened. There we were.

It had a crazy beginning but it ended on a good note.

We're lying in bed and then he was like, "Here's a picture of my kid." It was just a bad situation.

Mary, 22
Bronx, New York

TWO CAN PLAY THAT GAME
Kip, 23

I was 14, never met the girl before in my life. I talked on the phone with her for about two days, talked bullshit, whatever. My friend was trying to hook me up with her. It was kind of arranged which was the fucked-up part, and kind of made it uncomfortable.

End up going over to my friend's house and he and I both lost our virginities on the same night. Different girls, different rooms, but same night. He was raised by his grandfather so he had his run of the place. I'm chilling up in his grandfather's attic, met her, and lost my virginity to her that night. Probably the worst sex I've ever had. It was basically on a bare floor surrounded by spray-painted walls - tags me and my buddy put up there. My boy left two cigarettes up in the attic for him and I when we were done. He went downstairs, lost his virginity, came back up and we smoked. I never spoke to the girl again. Gave her a hug when she left his house. I fucking gave her a hug then sent her on her way.

The girl I slept with ended up going to school with us later on. She switched high schools and I ended up finding out that she had fucked half the people in my school. Then when I was like 18, 19, I found out she was doing low-class porn. So, interesting story, but not the best.

Honestly I wouldn't want to lose my virginity any other way except for a one-night stand. Otherwise you know how that goes, you get attached... *blah, blah, blah*... fuck that. I gave her a hug, peace, chucked the deuce up, "Later." Never talked to or saw her again until she transferred high schools. I don't think she cared either. She was probably into taking virginities. She was like on a warpath, taking virginities from what I later heard about her.

But here's the actual reason it went down the way it did, because my girlfriend at the time who was the same age as me, she went and cheated on me with some other guy and I come to find out that she lied about it and said that he raped her. Come to find out he didn't fucking rape her. She liked him, went to a fucking party with him and lost her virginity. He was like four years older than her.

I went and confronted the guy. I had a knife on me. I was going with the intent of hurting the guy. Instead he sat me down to talk with me and told me what really happened. Then one of my close friends told me that she walked in on them, which verified it so I was like, "Oh. All right, well fuck that. I'm going to get back at this bitch."

My buddy, the one who set us up with the girls, he was with me the night my girlfriend told me she was raped. So he decided to find girls we could have sex with so I could get revenge on my girlfriend.

We were actually still going out at the time and then as soon as I got it done I called her up and told her how I lost my virginity and she was so pissed off at me, which is sad because she cheated on me and lost her virginity to someone else first... but, oh man, talk about pissed off. That's how I broke up with her. Then she still tried to get back together with me. After all of that she still tried to get back together with me.

(...and how not to)

TELLING IT LIKE IT IS
Ramona, 28

It was with a sucker M.C. What led to it was my naïveté and my stupidity. But then again, it didn't come to anything because his dick was so small that I don't think that he did really anything.

When he was doing it, he was saying, "Whose pussy is it? Whose pussy is it?" And I was saying, "It's mine, it's mine." So he's a jerk... and he has a small dick.

I knew he was a loser, but to be quite honest I was tired of being a virgin and I wanted to just experience it. And on the real to real... I wasn't feeling him, and I guess he wasn't feeling me so that's why, overall, it wasn't good. Maybe if I would have been in love, and he would have been in love with me, it would've been another thing. But all it was was me being in a hurry to not be a virgin anymore and him being in a hurry to get in between my legs.

I waited almost two years before having another sexual experience because I did not enjoy the first one and I was like, "If that's the hype, I can do without." I really started enjoying it when I was 24, so it's like I could have waited until then.

Seriously, you've heard it before but I suggest you wait. Wait until you really feel something for that one person. Not just like, "Ooh, he's cute or I like his style or he dances real good or he's funny." No, no, no, no, no. I mean just feel that person in the true sense of it. And then you'll be able to enjoy your first experience. But if not, then it's a waste of your time and to be quite frank, pussy gets wrinkled, you know what I'm saying? Your parts get old. So if you don't keep yourself for the one person you want to share all your first experiences with then you're just gonna waste your body. It's like anything else. You wear shoes too much they get used – worn out. If you use your pussy too much, girlfriend, it's not gonna stay tight. And they don't like loose.

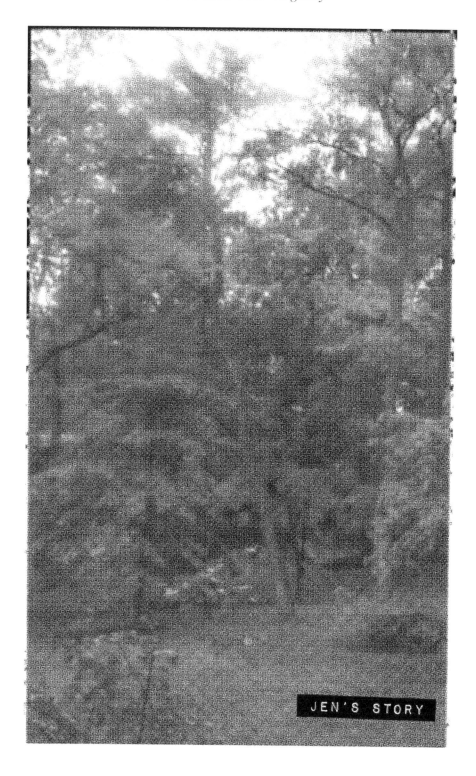

(...and how not to)

"NO MEANS NO."

12

Very early in the collection process I expected to eventually hear an account of a sexual assault. However, I was completely unprepared when it happened during interview 15, two weeks after I started the project. The first story in this chapter is number 15. These were the most difficult to listen to but I feel that, for these women, and men, they got the most in return for sharing their experiences. And they did so with a very real sense of empowerment in that, "This horrible thing happened to me but it must be told."

I feel that it is also important to note that many of those interviewed whose stories appear in this chapter stated that, given time and after some healing, they've gone on to healthy and fulfilling sex lives. That a tragic event hindered their sexual development and maturity, but it didn't arrest it completely.

The Rape Abuse & Incest National Network, RAINN, operates a National Sexual Assault Hotline, 24 hours a day at 1-800-656-HOPE (4673).

Or you can search for your local rape crisis center at http://www.rainn.org

PAM'S STORY
Pam, 41

My dad was in the hotel business, so I moved around a lot as a child. We were living in Chicago and at the time vacationing in a little town called Williams Bay, up in Wisconsin. In the summer months they have a little town festival with firemen shooting hoses at barrels up in the air. Stuff like that. Stan Kazowski was running one of the little carnival booths there. I just thought he was dreamy.

I met him again when he was out one night fishing on the pier behind where my parents and I were staying. He was obviously not supposed to be there. It was for our building, but he was pretty cute and he asked me out.

He was 19, I was almost 15. My parents knew I was going out with him and his father was the sheriff and they had his phone number so they must have thought I'd be safe. They didn't know there would be a car involved. That part was secret.

I walked three blocks to the town center where we met in a little park. He had a guy named Randall with him, who years later I'd still know. I still know Stan in a way; I obviously don't speak to him anymore. Anyway, they took me to the Thumbs Up bar in Lake Geneva, Wisconsin, where they served Michelob in Michelob glasses.

This was the first time I was in a car with a boy. First time I was ever in a bar. First time drinking save for sneaking a sip of my dad's scotch. For every beer I had in front of me there was two more waiting. I had never been drunk before. I thought that being drunk was like a thing, like you were sober and then you're drunk. I didn't know that you could get more drunk. I didn't know about falling down drunk. Didn't know about falling down the steep staircase to the bathroom drunk.

We left the bar, we were in his car. I'm talking about a ten-minute drive from one small town to another. He pulled over by the lake and this was the only time I had ever been that drunk, when you lose muscle control, when you're a puddle. I puke on me. I puke on him. I puke in the backseat. Somehow this is still gonna go down. I guess he couldn't break my hymen because I heard him tell me, "I'm gonna get this done no matter what." The next thing I knew it was over and I was in my own puke, in the backseat.

I got home at seven o'clock in the morning and my parents were furious. They screamed at me and I immediately got in the bathtub. They'd been on the phone with his sheriff dad all night.

The sheriff dad knew how old I was. I didn't hear anyone mention statutory rape and my parents just assumed I was in the wrong. Whether I had sex or not wasn't even discussed. It was my first date and I'd been out all night; that's all my parents needed to know.

I remember not understanding it. I didn't know I wasn't a virgin anymore because I was still thinking I was saving myself for marriage. I wrote in my journal that we were in love, that we were dating. My mother read it and when we got back to Chicago she made an appointment with the gynecologist to get "the pill". She went hysterical. I went down to my dad's office, he's the executive of the entire hotel, and I burst into tears. My father said, "Honey, think of the pill as insurance." My mom thought I was naughty and my daddy gave me carte blanche. So I turned into a tramp. It wasn't until I was in graduate school that I realized or even admitted to myself that I was raped. At least it was the '70s and I didn't get sick.

(...and how not to)

BOBBI'S STORY
Bobbi, 22

I was going over this friend's house to get high. We went over to this other guy's house instead. I think his name was Danny. Six hours later, I woke up without pants. That's my story.

    I don't know if my virginity was stolen. I don't know if it was consensual. I don't know 'cause I don't remember.

    I was pretty upset because before this happened I had anticipated the first time would be something special. After this happened it wasn't special anymore. I saw him one other time at school and I just walked away. After that I had a lot of sex because I stopped caring. It took me a long time to realize I should care. I was 15, no maybe 14.

    Looking back, I wish I had never got high. I wish it didn't have to happen the way it did. I probably would have been a virgin for a very, very long time 'cause, other than the drugs I was a good girl.

    I could have been in a blackout saying, "Yes." So, I don't know. It's a pretty steep accusation calling it rape if you're not sure so... don't do drugs. That's my advice.

HERBERT'S STORY
Herbert C, 82

It happened when I was young, with my brother. And in all respect, all gay people, it started with a cousin, or brother, or some shit. I will knock your socks off with this one. My brother, he was a drunk. We lived in the same room, my brother, my older brother, and a younger brother. And Arnold would go out and he would come home drunk and, I don't know if I wanted it, I didn't want it but he was drunk and he would make me take all my clothes off and he would hack off on me. Which, he was my brother, I would never say a fucking word about it to anyone.

    I never sucked his dick, but he would get on top of me and hack off. And after he hacked off he'd take off again and go drink some more. Now this went on and on and on. Then one night he came home, I don't know, maybe he was in a pissed-off mood. He was drunk. I was asleep in my bed and he crawled over me and stuck his prick right between my legs. I said, "Keep away from me." I said, "I love you. You're my brother." I got pissed off. I start yelling. My father came in and, "What's he doing?" "He's doing dirty things." My father took him, bent him over and with a strap, beat the fucking ass off him.

    Then again, maybe I started liking it and I used to look forward to it. Here I am today as gay as they make 'em. I'm 82 and I like prick. I love black, I love Spanish. I'll suck anybody clean.

MAC'S STORY
Mac, 46

In a place called Woodman Mobile Home Park near Ashtabula, Ohio, that's where I grew up. My mom was an alcoholic – a barmaid. And the neighbors – two girls, they always abused me – beat me up. This was abuse, boy I'll tell you. I got scars on my back still, cigarette marks.

These girls were my babysitters. My mom would go to work and these girls would sit there and get me all worked up and then they threw me out of the damn trailer in the wintertime and then they'd take me back in and tie me up. They really liked to play with your head. They were sick like that.

I was just a kid and hell, one was a senior. The other one was like in 10th grade and I was... shit, in sixth grade. Oh, they were sick bitches. One was a real fat-ass. They'd ask favors to go do this and do that. But it was them messing with your head. It got to the point where you think you did something right and then all of a sudden you're getting your ass whooped. If I did something wrong they'd tie me up.

I told my mother the story and she took me to the doctor. She thought I had a problem, making up stories like that. Who could come up with those bizarre stories? This went on for about a year and a half. Then the one girl got cancer and her family moved to New York to get special treatment at some hospital. And that's when it stopped. That's what saved me because that broke up their little party when the one left, she was sick in the head more than the one who stayed. Matter of fact, I saw the sick bitch about four years ago working in some damn gas station back home. And she recognized who I was too. Man, I was ready to go kick her damn ass. It wasn't fun what they did to me. It sucked. It messed with your head and as soon as you didn't play their game you got your ass beat.

It was like sex was good, but not the way they were doing it. I actually got off the first time and she was on me, rubbing me, shit like that, trying to get off, and then they'd beat the hell out of me. Turned the whole damn thing around. Actually I was getting off and... "Whoa. I think she stabbed me or something." You know what I mean? Stuff coming out of me, like what the hell happened?

I'd have sex with both of them and they used to laugh all the time about it, about getting naked and shit with me. Then they were doing each other. I mean, I'm a kid, you know? I didn't have pubes. When I told my mother about how they would beat the shit out of me, oh my god, she looked at me like I was an idiot. Like, Jesus Christ, who'd make that one up?

But yeah, my mother worked at a bar. She was an alcoholic. That was a fucked-up life. It's hard to deal with women now. These girls were my neighbors. One lived on one side, the other lived on the other side. Jesus Christ, I was in the middle.

Friends of mine, they thought I was off the wall. They didn't have those hidden cameras back then or little tape recording pens, you know? So all the bizarre shit they did and the more I told, the more idiotic I looked.

They'd laugh and shit, "Oh, you got a little hardon. You're not gonna tell your mom. You're not gonna or we'll kick your ass," then they'd tie me up and start playing with me and shit. That messed my head up.

(...and how not to)

And I knew what was going on. Well, kind of I knew. I hung with boys so, at that age you always talked about it. I told these guys and even they didn't believe me. But these girls were good. They knew everyone would think I was a nut if I talked about it. Nobody believed that shit. But I still got the cigarette marks on my back to prove it. I didn't make those up. If I didn't listen or do what they wanted then I got that domination shit.

You know, speaking of the cigarette burns, I was like, "Mom, look at this." I still don't know how they got out of that one. They turned it into me messing around with something and me getting hurt. You know, they turned everything around. Like at first I thought it was cool and I told my best friend about it, but then the girls they started sticking me with pins and burning my damn back.

That's a sick way for a kid. But that's how I busted the 'ole cherry. I don't know... hey, top that one, huh?

JEN'S STORY
Jen, 22

I was 15 and hanging at our local mall. When you left the first level you could walk across the parking lot to another little strip mall. At the time there was this field with a bunch of trees and everything in the center. It was three o'clock in the afternoon and I was walking from the mall, down the block to my boyfriend's house and I was jumped from behind by two guys. They knocked me out and I woke up ass naked in the middle of that field. It wasn't even a big, secluded area. It was just, you know, some trees and bushes and stuff.

They came at me from behind and *whack*. I only know there were two of them because I caught them from behind, just a quick glance before they attacked me from behind the trees. I don't remember any of it. I picked up my clothes, got dressed, and continued on to my boyfriend's house like nothing happened.

I didn't tell anyone for a couple years. I was too embarrassed, too ashamed. That was seven years ago. I was young and back then we just didn't talk about it.

I don't think I had a concussion because I didn't throw up or anything, even though I was hit in the head a bunch of times. It wasn't a concussion but I was definitely knocked out for a bit. Physically, I felt it for a few days afterward and emotionally I was hurt for a long time after that.

I was too embarrassed and too ashamed to go to the hospital. I just kept the whole thing to myself. My boyfriend didn't question me. He just figured I was hanging out at the mall a little bit longer than I planned.

I wasn't able to talk about it until I was raped again when I was 18. So much bad shit has happened. Fuck it. You can't change it. I'm not going to be miserable because of it.

I was hanging out with people I shouldn't have been. I had just gotten out of a mental hospital that my mom put me in when we were fighting. She thought I was going crazy so she went through like seven doctors to get me committed. Then she went through six hospitals to find me a bed. When I got out I went to a party and that happens to me again.

Ah... I've been through so much shit. Fuck it. Life sucks. It goes on.

CARLA'S STORY
Carla Q, 30

CARLA Q: I lost my virginity when I was two or three.

SHAWN WICKENS: A family member?

CQ: Who cares? I was adopted. This is how it goes... anyways... so I got cancer now. The Huntsman Cancer Institute, you know that man Jon Huntsman?

SW: Not really.

CQ: Big money in Utah. Jon Huntsman, you know the cancer center? They want to do a study on my ass because you know what? I got cancer 'cause from all the fucking... that's why I got cervical cancer now, from scar tissue and abuse.

SW: This was repeated abuse over time?

CQ: Uh-huh. And I got... I'm 30 now. I was 21 when they diagnosed me.

SW: Are you in remission now?

CQ: Hell no, I'm sicker than it gets.

SW: So you don't remember who it was...

CQ: I know exactly who it was. The fucker that bought me. But what does it matter you see, 'cause I'm in Salt Lake City, Utah. And the state of Utah took custody of me out of... I was out of Baltimore, out of DC. I was a fucking six-inch fucking scarecrow with fucking these liberty spikes, boom-boom I've been on the streets since I was 10 and off and on and then again, and then Utah took custody of me, brought me the fuck here.

Some people don't lose their virginity, they just get raped or robbed or fucking...

SW: Did that give you sort of a skewed view of sex, because of your introduction of it?

CQ: Up until now, probably, but not now. Like this, I've never been a hooker. I've never been a whore. I've fuckin' gone on the streets and said, "Fuck this shit. I ain't gonna sell my body for nuthin'." But fuckin' runned it and gunned it and fuckin' stole dope and shit. But it ain't like I've been with a bunch of fuckin' motherfuckers since. Yes, it skewed my perception but you know what, once when I got with somebody that I had made love with then I knew the difference. Like that. But, what's a fucking virgin, you know? A sin is a sin is a sin, you know what I mean? I lost my virginity when I was 3 maybe when I was 30. Shit. Impress me, maybe I'll lose it again.

SW: Anything else?

(...and how not to)

CQ: Zip-zap, you're in the wrong state. Tat for a tat.

Let me tell you when I lost my virginity to a woman. Carla here wants to talk about the bisexualness of fucking... It got quiet in the bar, let me wait a minute.

When I was a shy guy, too. I made love to a woman... I did it. I said I made love to a woman but I was missing the dick... didn't get the prick. That's all good 'cause at the time I wasn't looking for the stick. And that's why those little ladies over there have some massive gaydar on me, right now. They're giving me the fucking flame, you know, and I know every one of their names and I don't give a fuck, Chuck. 'Cause I already fucking pigeoned the duck. I'm feeding you your need, I'm giving you your dope, you know what I'm saying, 'cause shit, none of us say, fuckin' let's hang on a rope.

So here's the story. So I was like, I'm sick of these men these pricks and shit, ever since I was locked up in Baltimore. I'm talking about the ponytail... I'm locked in Baltimore... So I'm like, fuck all this shit, right? I was locked down. There was like 150-250 bitches in there, ain't a fucking dude around. It wasn't even like that, that's the way I learned to love. Where it's safe and shit, where you got your little best friend buddy.

Then after I got out I was with this woman for like six years so I had to live loud and proud in Salt Lake City, Utah, with her and her little boy, you know what I'm saying? And people are ignorant. We'd be driving, "Hey you fucking dykes, you bitches..." you know what I'm saying? I got a son in the back of my car. What are you talking about, you know what I'm saying? I been in places, shit... Evanston, Wyoming, isn't far from here where they killed that fucking boy... and strung him to the fucking fence.

SW: Matthew Shepard?

CQ: Hell yeah. Exactly. Straight up. So it's not like I don't live with a constant awareness that I went from fucking being fucking raped to getting fucking fucked on all the time. Then I was with a woman and I was handling my shit, and these motherfuckers that get so goddamned ignorant and you're like, "Fuck, it's not even safe to be fucking..." 'Cause I ain't no fucking scrub. I know what's up.

I'm in charge of my own sex life now... and I have a great sex life, for sure, now. But it's like 12 years later and it took 10 years for me to enjoy sex. And... that guy was a goddamn bastard for sure.

Wendy, 26
Madison, Wisconsin

NICOLAS'S SIDE OF THE STORY
Nicolas, 34

This was in middle school. This was like... ninth grade. I met this girl through my cousin and I thought I was straight at the time, at least I was trying to live like I was straight. She had a quality about her that I thought was sensual and welcoming. I was living with my grandmother and at my grandmother's house you could sneak up the back way, like on different roofs to get into my room. I got her to come around one night to the other side of the house and climb up the roofs and from there, there was this pole you could climb up and then jump on the roof and then jump in the window.

We were friends since I guess we were 10 but her father didn't want me to date her. He always gave me this like disapproving expression on his face. Her father always disapproved of me and I never understood why until years later when my cousin told me, "He always thought you were gay and that you would be bad for his daughter because you wouldn't give her the love she deserved." But I was like, "She was young too. What kind of love could I give her?"

But anyway, he knew I was gay and he was right. And I always saw her father as beautiful, like this quintessential male and I respected him so much because I thought he was noble. But he never accepted me. Anyway, his daughter and I dated and she snuck into my bedroom and we had sex and she started crying, which my first thought with my perverted sort of closeted gay male sensibilities was like, "Oh she's crying because I'm a man, and I'm hurting her, and I'm penetrating her, and maybe it's her first time." It wasn't her first time, it was my first time. I should've been crying too, because the reason she was crying was because she felt like I forced her into having sex. But I didn't even realize that I forced her. But if that's how she felt then I guess I did force her. How could I deny that if that's what she felt? And she was crying because she was so disappointed with the situation.

We hadn't talked about having sex, it was all just nonverbal communication. It was basically me helping her through the window, and you know like, "Oh this is bad but good at the same time." And then we were lying on my bed and everything went from there. It was all sort of nonverbal. I took off her pants, then I took off my pants. But strangely enough we both had our tops on. I was erect and I tried to penetrate her and it wasn't working. I wasn't experienced. I didn't think she was either but later she told me she was.

She was unhappy with how everything went down. I'm thinking she's a virgin and I penetrated her, that must hurt and, "Oh, what a man I must be." And it had nothing to do with that. She was completely utterly disgusted with me because she didn't want to have sex with me in that way, sneaking through my bedroom window, any of it.

Her and I never reconciled; we hardly even looked at each other afterwards. It was always avoidance. Constant avoidance but for different reasons. I thought she was avoiding me because we had sex. But she was really avoiding me because she felt I raped her. But she never let me know like, "Oh, Nicolas this is not right." I was thinking, hoping, it was sort of an overwhelming kind of spiritual thing for her but it had nothing to do with that. It was disappointment and disgust and anger towards me.

(...and how not to)

AMANDA'S STORY
Amanda, 23

I met River at a coffee shop. Cup of Joe's Garage was the cool hangout in the town I grew up in near San Diego. I was the typical insecure girl and he was older and intellectual and different. And he was interested in me. We hung out for a couple of months and got to know each other, became friends. Then he started to really dig me and he started to do all these sweet, nice things. He made me tapes with songs on them and he wrote me poetry.

We were at his mom's apartment where he still lived, in his room, and he gave me some beer. I never had beer before and I got drunk. It was a date rape situation. And then afterwards he pretty much abandoned me. He didn't talk to me, didn't call me and I was very confused by that. It was my first experience with alcohol and my first experience with sex and because of that experience, for the next five years of my life I thought sex was about me lying on my back until the man was finished.

I don't spend much time in my hometown now, but I went back years later and I saw him, and somewhat confronted him and said, "You'll never know..." in a nice way, "You'll never know what an effect you had on my life." And I didn't clarify negative or positive... but it was negative. Maybe positive, maybe it opened my eyes to somewhat the true nature of some men. But he gave me some random, intellectual comment or quote and I said, "Yeah, River. You're so deep." And I just walked away and I felt so good.

Yeah. There was like half a dozen girls in our town that he did this to. That was his tactic. Play the part of the intellectual, find a naïve girl and make them believe he really liked them. Then he'd get them drunk, took what he wanted from them, and then never spoke to them again. There had to have been six girls who I knew personally that he had taken their virginity. He was an evil bastard. I was 15.

> I definitely see how it's affected me in later years. And since it was the babysitter who molested me... it forced me to become more distrustful of authority figures.
>
> *Frank, 29*
> *Philadelphia, Pennsylvania*

How to Lose Your Virginity

HENRY'S STORY
Henry, 48

I was seven and it was with my cousin through marriage. I know it's fucked up but that's how it happened. Happened while my Aunt Bernadette's daughter, Sandra, was babysitting me. Now I have a real aversion to heavyset women because of two incidents, the losing of my virginity and one other one.

The first incident was when I was five. My mom was white, it was an interracial marriage. She was from Montana and my dad was from Mississippi. When we used to go to Baptist churches it was like my brother and I were on display because our mother was white.

This one Sunday we're in the back of Scott's Methodist Church, sitting in a pew. This lady comes over sits in the space next to me. I'll never forget this, she had a light purple dress on and she's all of 350 lbs.... all of 350. This is in an evangelistic church and they had nurses and stuff to fan people who got the Holy Ghost and fainted. So I'm sitting and the big lady's sitting right next to me. All of a sudden she gets the Holy Ghost in her. She jumps up and throws her arms back and hits me in the nose. I fall into the corner of the pew and she falls down on top of me. Nobody knows I'm up under her because she's all of 350 lbs.

If you're ever been to an evangelistic church, the music is going, the preacher is going... it's chaotic! I'm under there and she's got a girdle on so she can't feel me under there. Pretty soon she sees blood, she thinks she's bleeding and panics. My mother grabs my brother because she thinks I'm missing. Finally they get her off me, but not before I'm feeling abandoned by females because my mom didn't save me from up under this great big weight.

Then when I'm 7 or 8 my cousin Sandra was babysitting me and she's huge, big. And she used me to have sex with her on the bathroom toilet. I'm a kid, she's 18 and the only way she can get serviced is having me, her little cousin, sit on her. But I didn't even realize that what she did was wrong until my mid-40s.

I was watching that movie *Antoine Fisher*. I see the part in the movie when the lady who adopts Antoine starts slapping him around and I have an anxiety attack right in the theatre. It was almost like the same thing I went through because when my cousin wanted to do it and I wouldn't go along with her, she would get aggressive on me. When I was growing up I thought I was the shit because none of my friends my age were getting pussy. But at the same time, I now have a hard time with relationships and it wasn't until I was sitting in the theatre and I saw it happen on screen that I realized that.

I run an escort service and it's like I have an understanding of their sexuality, like I can relate to their whole well-being. I'd have to say that the females I work with, it's sad but probably 95% of them were molested as children. Most little kids who get taken advantage of are cute kids. That's just how it is. And back then I was considered exotic at the time... there weren't a lot of interracial marriages or products of interracial marriages. And I didn't even realize how fucked up what I went through was until I saw some similar exploitation in a movie. It overwhelmed me to the point where I had to be helped out of the theater, like I had gotten the Holy Ghost in me and passed out.

(...and how not to)

AILEEN'S STORY
Aileen K, 40

SHAWN WICKENS: Tell me about the first time.

AILEEN K: I don't need to say my name or anything, right? Uh... let's see... I--uh... Denise was my friend at the time and she still is.

SW: Right.

AK: At the time I was 14, eighth grade... and I was dating a guy named Hal.

SW: All right.

AK: And... Denise stop getting upset whenever I tell this story. And... uh, these boys said to us, "Let's relax, let's relax, let's relax."

SW: Where were you?

DENISE: In Englewood.

AK: We were at... no, not in Englewood. We were in Woodcliff Lake, New Jersey.

SW: OK.

AK: And he said, "Let's relax." And he gave us...

SW: You were at a house party?

AK: No...

D: It was in the basement of Hal's house.

AK: It was two boys, two girls.

SW: OK.

D: And he gave us Valium that was his grandmother's.

AK: His grandmother's Valium. I was on Valium. And that's when it happened... and I was in a back room. And I still had my shirt on... and I mean – I had my pants off, but I had my shirt on.

D: And I remember your expression after it happened.

AK: The first time… you don't want your shirt on. You want your shirt off. You want it to be like intense and everything. And… I just remember him struggling a little bit to get it in and then him struggling to get it out. And it was not fun at all. And like I said I had my shirt on. So it was all about, you know, the sex of it all. And I came outside and… and I came outside and my best friend, Denise, was standing there…

SW: Right.

AK: Waiting for me outside and what did you… Denise, come here. You have to verbalize it. You have to verbalize it…

SW: Denise, were you at all drugged up as Aileen was?

D: I was drugged up but I… I fell asleep. And when I woke up she was standing there with her hands folded in front of her with a real foul look on her face, and I said, "What happened?" And that's when she said, "I had sex with him." And I'll never forget that look on her face as long as I live.

AK: And the only thing that I remember that I was really disappointed in was… number one, I was too young. I wanted the love and I wanted the hugs, the kisses. I didn't want the fucking penetration. And the other thing is, my shirt was on.

SW: What… what effect did the drugs have on you? Did you pass out or you just couldn't move or anything? I've never done Valium…

AK: Valium makes you sleepy.

D: Valium. It was Valium. And I remember it was 10mg a pill and he gave us two each. I fell asleep. He raped you.

AK: Oh, so… yeah it was considered rape, if you think about it. Date rape, maybe, possibly. Um… it just left me very relaxed and very sleepy.

SW: Right.

AK: I was not ready for the intercourse thing, I was just ready for… I was ready for a boyfriend, but not for that.

SW: Did you break up with him soon after that? Did you stop seeing him…

AK: Oh, yeah. He wanted a girlfriend with long red nails (laughs). I can laugh about it now, 'cause it's funny. He said he wanted a girlfriend with long red nails.

D: I'll never laugh about it… 'cause I'll remember your expression standing there in the semi-darkness, with your hands folded in front of you and tears in your eyes. I don't find it anything funny to laugh about it.

AK: Yeah. That's my best friend. That's my best friend.

(...and how not to)

SW: How soon after it happened... 'cause earlier you said your mother knows. How... when did you tell her about it?

AK: Oh, god... let's see. Hang on a second. This happened like spring, and then in summer I became like a slut because... once a teenager... no, no, no. Seriously, once a teenager loses it they become a slut. Bottom line. I am not ashamed of that. My mother knows everything. I am not ashamed of it.

D: You weren't a slut.

AK: No, not a slut. I was... I was free. And what happened was... my mother found out. I would say in September.

SW: Right.

AK: It happened in April... my mother found out everything in September.

SW: And what did she say?

AK: Oh my god. I came home, well she... it's a long story.

SW: Right.

AK: OK... Hang on, my mother, no... it was my stepmother who read my diary. And she went and told my mother, I came home from track one day, and my mother just said, "You! You! You! I read your diary! Oh my god. Oh my god!"

D: I remember that. And you were running down my street, screaming, crying. And your brother Scott was in the car following behind you.

AK: You know the movie *Thirteen*? You know, it's similar to that. I can understand the movie *Thirteen*. Mine was all... I mean, I didn't do all those drugs but I did a lot of the alcohol. And girls don't really...

D: Bad memories for me. You losing your virginity. Bad memories.

AK: Look at her, she's upset. Denise, Denise, yours wasn't so dramatic though.

SW: Were you upset about Aileen so much though 'cause you... I mean was there a feeling that you got off easy in a way, 'cause you were drugged too, and sort of nothing happened?

D: I fell asleep so I felt like I wasn't there to protect her. That's what I felt like. I was 18 when I lost my virginity. So I was out of high school. But for her I felt like... I fell asleep and I let her down.

SW: Where did the other guy go that was also there?

D: He fell asleep too.

AK: I don't think he took Valium. I think he was smoking pot or something. Yeah. But I really want teenagers, teenage girls in the world to hear something like this.

SW: Of course, because it happens. It happens.

AK: Um… after that, I have to say after a teenager, after a teenage girl or a pre-teen girl goes through something like that… they long and long and long and long for more. But I don't think it's sex they want. It's intimacy they want. It's not sex. They think they want sex. But it's not. They want intimacy. They think the sex makes up for it. That's why when I saw the movie, *Thirteen,* I was like, "Oh my god." Like I wasn't that bad… but it was… it… it affected me when I saw that movie.

(...and how not to)

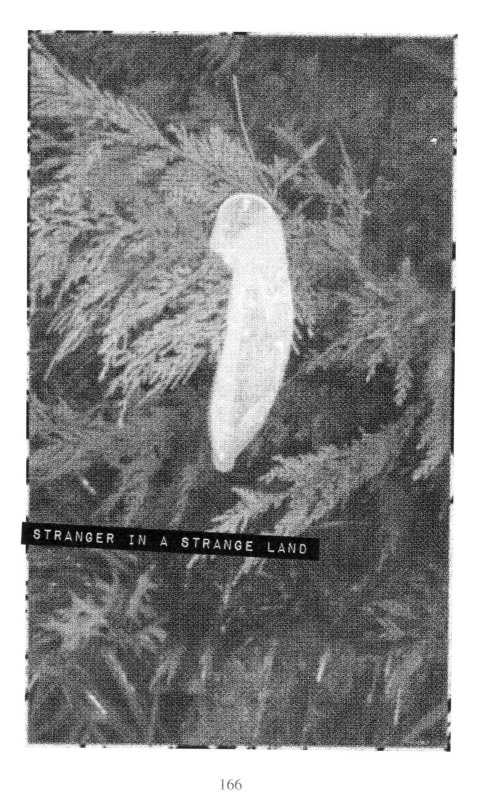

(...and how not to)

"THAT'S ME IN THE SPOTLIGHT, LOSING MY RELIGION"

13

I was taught at a very early age, from parents, school, and church that premarital sex was a sin, that you had to wait for marriage. And while the bishop in my hometown would announce a special dispensation allowing for Catholics to eat corned beef when St. Patrick's Day happened to fall on a Friday during Lent, there exists no dispensation for sex before marriage. Some rules can be bent, others not. And growing up in a religious family was a source for some internal conflict, while pre-marital sex was handled with such severity and absolute consequences with the church, it was dealt with so casually in the secular world.

Waiting for marriage is a main component to several other religions. And it wasn't until I spoke with Betsy from Salt Lake City that I heard that Mormons believe premarital sex to be the most serious sin after murder. There's quite a difference between a biological urge and the taking of someone's life, but some people grew up unable to separate sex and feelings of guilt. There were those who were able to come to terms with it. But if you grew up with religion in your life, it's something you had to deal with at some point, or even repress completely.

TAKE OFF YOUR RING FIRST
Junger, 26

My uncle, my mom's brother, was doing some AIDS-related work throughout Africa. This one year for Christmas he gave my dad and I these shirts for an African condom company along with some condoms from that brand. My parents are pretty liberal so it was no big deal. The condoms ended up in a junk drawer with like pens and paper and who knows what else.

I had been dating the same girl all through high school, or at least my junior and senior years. I thought I was in love, thought I was probably going to marry her. But she was this major Christian girl and she had this promise ring that her parents had given her signifying she wouldn't have sex before she got married. She wore that tiny ring on a necklace either to appease her folks or herself, or maybe even to remind me, I don't know. It was weird. I wasn't a fan of that promise ring.

The summer before I went to college, like that June or July, she said, "Yeah, we should do it." I was like, "OK," so I had to rifle through the junk drawer to find one of the African condoms my uncle gave us as Christmas presents.

She ended up telling her dad about it and she told me her dad cried about it. I don't know if it was a guilt trip thing but she tried to lay it all on me about how upset he was and how he cried.

RECONCILIATION: FACE TO FACE
Marie, 25

My senior year of high school, I was 18 so I was legal per se. I was a volunteer with the EMS in my hometown in New Jersey, answering 911 calls, that sort of thing.

There was a party for the "New Squad", all the high school kids who volunteered with the ambulance corps. I got drunk, got completely annihilated and was there after everybody left 'cause I couldn't drive home.

It's just me and the host, this guy I worked with who was in his 30s. He starts giving me more drinks, and more drinks. He does the cheesy backrub thing. Next thing I know we're in his bed having sex. I was watching the clock the whole time. For a whole hour I was watching the clock. Finally at four in the morning I said, "I have school tomorrow and I have to get home before my parents notice I'm gone."

I get home and take a shower and I broke down. I couldn't believe I did such the cliché, have-sex-when-I'm-drunk, idiotic first time. It's so *After School Special*, but everyone does that. I told my best friend who said I should have a three-day grace period. "For three days you can vent and bitch and cry and moan. But after those three days if you're still upset, you gotta go see a professional." I'm like, "Fine." Three days later I was still so upset. I'm Catholic so I went to confession.

I was very big into the church. I had been an altar server, I was a Eucharistic minister, I was there every Sunday. I went to the rectory, pounded on the door totally bawling and found this priest I had known all my life and was like, "I need to talk to you."

(...and how not to)

    We sat down in his office, I'm on the couch and he's sitting in a recliner. Totally nonchalant, I'm wearing jeans, a t-shirt, and flip-flops. I tell him what happened and he was like, "Were you safe about it?" I said, "Yeah, we used a condom." He said, "OK. That's good." Which I thought was weird because the Catholic Church totally does not advocate condoms. Then the priest asked if the guy called the next day. "Um... well, no." "Oh, what a douche bag." I was like, "What? What did you say?" He said, "The guy should call the next day. I'm really sorry, Marie." Then he told me it was good I admitted it, that it wasn't the end of the world, and that it'll make me stronger. He sent me on my way without a penance. The whole thing was odd but sort of euphoric. I felt cleansed.

    The guy did end up calling me a day later. I lied and told him everything was OK. We had been friends, but it was never the same between us. We never really talked again and sometime later he moved out West and got married.

    I got over it and was like, "All right, whatever. Guys suck." Soon after that I decided I was gay and that ended that. Later I found out from most of my girlfriends that their first times were horrifying too, and pretty much everyone cried afterwards.

    One of the other volunteers ended up asking me what happened after everyone left the party. She was like, "We knew something was going to happen. That's why we all left." Gee, thanks.

THE HOLY GRAIL
Dorothy, 39

I waited until I was 29. I waited because of religious beliefs and I was clinging to that. I was really struggling with whether I believed it or not and this was the last thing that I was clinging to as proof that I still believed.

    After I started falling away from my religious beliefs, it was getting kind of embarrassing and I was at the point were I couldn't admit it to people I was dating because it was just weird. The person who was the one, I told him I was a virgin and he said it didn't matter. It didn't matter whether I did or didn't. That sort of gave me permission to be fine with it.

    We had been dating for three months when it actually happened and it was kind of an accident. He asked me if I wanted to, and I said, "Yes," meaning in the future or at a later date. And he's like, "Ok, let me go get a condom." I was just like, "OK. All right. It's gonna be now," and I decided to go along with it.

    It was a fairly different situation with most people because it was so weighted for me. It had become such a big thing in my mind because I felt so much older than average. But maybe I wasn't hurt in the way that other people have been who jump into something that's purely physical. In retrospect I might have done it differently. But I think that people take the step whenever they're ready. You can't really second guess yourself as to where you are... because that's where you are.

BASIC TRAINING
Jonas, 28

I'd held off for a lot of years, had a couple of chances but because of my Mormon upbringing I always backed off at the point of penetration. It didn't occur until I got into the military. I was studying Russian at the Defense Language Institute and after being there for six months, a hot chick finally transferred into our unit.

Everybody else got really sort of aggressive on her and for whatever reason I just held off and played hard to get. Because of that and maybe she could smell my virginity and innocence, she singled me out. I thought I was in control, but I later realized she was playing me the entire time. She was very experienced. After our second date, that was it. We were in the midst of the usual makeout session I was conditioned to, traditionally involved in, where everything stopped before it went too far. But she was a little more active and engaged and because she was a pro she drew me out of the reasons I had resisted women before.

It didn't last long, we're talking 17 seconds. At first I felt shock that I actually went through with it. I got up, pulled away and was like, "Oh, God. You don't understand. I'm Mormon." I told her that I had been holding off until marriage because otherwise it's an unforgivable sin.

Not more than a minute after it happened I left her on the bunk bed and I went in the bathroom to sit on the toilet with my head in my hands. She was actually quite sweet about it. She pulled me back into bed and basically ended up nurturing me. She laid me down and stroked my head and spent the next half hour telling me it was perfectly natural, completely normal, completely acceptable, and that everything was all right. I didn't believe it then, but the next morning when I woke up I started to recall her comfort and the way she sort of placated me, and I ended up coming through it pretty guilt-free.

A certain part of me, for many years after that, resented her because I allowed myself to go against my faith and my religion and my ethics. But she definitely opened my eyes and both delicately and gently introduced me to a new world and did it with such finesse that the next time I was with a woman, I was in love and prepared for that intimate moment. The guilt didn't hold me back from the next relationship and it was really rewarding because of that first woman. I never even realized it until speaking about it now, but goddamn for years I hated that girl, and goddamn I'm really thankful for her.

> We drove up to the gate and it was closed. We were locked in on the grounds of the seminary and we both thought that it was a sign from God telling us we did something wrong and we could never leave.
>
> *Amber, 38*
> *Warwick Neck, Rhode Island*

(...and how not to)

MISSIONARY
Peter, 23

When I was still in college I went on a summer missionary trip to Kenya. I was working with two priests and a handful of other students from my school, which I'm not going to name, in a little village outside of Nairobi. Every day we would bring in kids from the secondary school. I helped with the choir because I was involved with the theater in high school and college. This one choir girl, I'll call her Mary, had a great voice. She was 16. I was 19 at the time and we started hanging out outside of the church. I met her family and stuff like that. We would just hang out, go for long walks; we just had a good time together.

One night we were in her room just practicing choir, nothing out of the ordinary but that's when it happened. We hadn't even kissed before then, but she kissed me and we started making out and then it went further and further. She hadn't had sex before either.

I did have a condom on me because I had been brought up in a public school environment with condoms ingrained in my head. So I had them with me not because I intended on having sex but because you never know. When I knew I was going to her house that night I brought one with me.

There were three other students with me on this trip, two girls and one gay guy. I didn't really feel comfortable with any of them keeping my confidence so I didn't tell anyone and I especially had to keep it secret from the priests. They would not have approved of the relationship, let alone me having condoms on the trip.

Mary told her brother and he was surprisingly OK with it. So as far as I knew he was the only other person who found out about it until I got back to the States. And I still haven't told many people. I told my best friends, I told my brothers and sister. It's not like the best story to tell. But that's what we did.

We had sex a few more times and continued to, I guess, like date. But in that environment it wasn't really dating. We couldn't go out on dates; it was more her coming for choir practice and then me walking her home. She came into my room a couple times which we were definitely not allowed to do. There was a strict "no guest" rule in our rooms, guys or girls. So those were the risky times but when I was over her house her parents trusted me 100%. The door was closed and it was no problem.

I think her brother was expecting a longer-term relationship. Her brother was expecting for me to take care of her and I kind of avoided that, made it as little of an issue as I could. But Mary knew I was going home so I think her expectations were low for that sort of thing. Obviously her parents didn't know about it otherwise I'm sure that would've been a huge thing. I mean, they were a family from the Catholic parish in their village so it would have been bad.

But Mary was a great girl. I've never talked to her or written her since even though we exchanged addresses. She hasn't contacted me either. It was nice for what it was. She was happy with it. I was happy with it. At no point did I feel like I was violating her.

CATCH-22
Don, 41

I was 21, kind of older for losing your virginity. I was in college at Texas A&M, big football school. This girl picked me up at a bar and unbeknownst to me she was dating a football player.

Went back to her place and we were enjoying ourselves. That night was the best of both worlds, it was the greatest and the worst experience of my life. We ended up in her room having sex and everything and I was all nervous and all of a sudden a bunch of people come over to her place so there's this huge party going on downstairs. Everybody's drinking and doing shots, and then her football player boyfriend shows up.

He was coming to her door which snapped me back to reality after such a blissful moment. I was grabbing for my clothes, wanting to hightail it out of there because the guy was bigger than I was. And in my immaturity, I wanted to prove to my friends that I'd gotten laid so in one fell swoop I grabbed her panties, left my clothes, jumped out her window and ran naked all the way back to my dorm room.

I didn't get caught. It was a clean getaway, I just had a bruised ego. We finished, I thought I was a stud and then seconds later I was just another guy running for his life, naked. I don't think the boyfriend ever found out about it. I'm not sure because that was the one and only time I ever saw or talked to that girl. So it wasn't like a loving or emotional thing it was more just like an animalistic act.

I proudly displayed the panties for my friends when I got back, but then I immediately called my younger sister to tell her I lost my virginity and that I was going to hell. I just needed to talk to somebody who understood that I kind of felt fucked up. After the initial thrill of it, I became so guilt ridden. I was raised Catholic, that's why I waited so long. On the one hand I didn't really care about it, but on the other hand I was like, "Oh my God, I've committed a mortal sin. That's been 20 years ago now and I'm doing all right.

BAPTISED IN THE RIVER
Fran, 28

I was in the Ogeechee River, in Georgia. My family had a river house so we would go there in the summertime and spend the night and have parties and stuff like that, although we weren't supposed to be there, boys and girls together... we all were.

My boyfriend and I, we were playing around, and I was on his hips in the water. He got aroused and we were already in the vicinity. It was kind of like, "I'll just put it in a little bit." And then a little bit more became a little bit more. And a little bit more. It happened right in the river when I was 14. He was 15. We were each other's firsts.

I got little upset because I thought I was going to burn in hell. And then I kind of thought, "Well, we already kinda did it, we might as well have sex again." And I only felt guilty for about a week so we did it again, full on, on the top bunk of the river house.

And just a little twist on the story, he also had an artificial leg. He lost it to bone cancer. That made for interesting sex.

(...and how not to)

THE VOW OF CHASTITY
Oscar, 34

I had notions of becoming a priest or joining one of the Catholic orders so I held off and I stayed a virgin up until I was 25. I was in a discernment program and I was doing weekly stints at a seminary in Baltimore. I had met and spoken with archbishops about taking my vows so I was very close to going through with it. And the average age of men entering the seminary is like 28, 28 to 32. It's a lot older these days so 25 was around the prime age.

Ultimately I decided that the priesthood was not for me and that I had no intentions of getting married so I decided I should enjoy my youth while I still had some. Luckily I hooked up with this girl who was an old grade school buddy; we used to ride the bus together. Lani knew all my history, knew my past, knew there were no skeletons in the closet. We weren't in love so that was good. She was a nurse so she explained everything to me in detail, what was going to happen, all the potential risks.

She was doing a nursing stint in Memphis and I was at her apartment visiting for a weekend. I sat her down and I was like, "Lani, would you be willing to share my virginity with me?" She said yes and that she would be honored.

Before the deed, I was getting ready for bed and brushing my teeth, looking in the mirror and thinking, "Oh my god, this is ridiculous. I'm 25 and I'm having this goddamn moment." But it went really smooth and great and this is gonna sound silly, but at the end of it she started to cry. I was like, "Why are you crying?" And she said, "I thought you said you were a virgin." I'm like, "I am a virgin!" She was like, "Then how did you learn to have sex so good?" I was like, "I'm a natural? I don't know."

But she was crying because she thought I lied about being a virgin to get her into bed. We talked again and I reassured her that she was my first. It set a good tone of honesty and me being down-to-earth about sex with later partners. I feel happy that I've kind of continued that throughout my sexual history. Maybe waiting a long time for reasons other than you can't get laid makes you be able to appreciate it a little bit more when the time finally comes.

It was funny because like I said we weren't in love but after having sex I thought I was in love with her. And she said, "Nah... that's just the sex." So I went back home and after a little while I slept with another girl and I called up Lani and I told her, "Yeah, you were right it was... it was the sex."

> As we're getting into things the alarm clock radio in the hotel room goes off and it's really, really loud music, "Jesus loves you, yes he does." It's about one or two in the morning, we're doing it, and this Christian Gospel radio station is blaring Jesus music at us. It was traumatic. It's playing on the other side of the room and you don't want to stop right away, but then you didn't want to hear that reminder that you're sinning either.
>
> *Margot, 24*
> *Cleveland, Ohio*

CULTURE SHOCK
Rushdy, 29

I was in high school... this was in Egypt. And we should be studying for our last year in school as it was a very hard year. Suad was maybe five or six years older than us. She used to be married and then she came back home to stay with her family. We found out later that she was divorced. It's not as bad as it used to be but it's still unusual to be divorced.

We knew her from a long time earlier. Three years earlier we used to know guys who would sleep with her but not break her virginity at all. I don't know if some people understand how you can sleep with a woman and not touch her... just like just outside the bodies, without the whole connection – clothes on.. She had to be scared to lose her virginity because when she got married if the husband find out that she had lost her virginity it's a big problem. She would be divorced the next day and then she would get killed from her family the day after that. So it's kind of complicated.

Actually she pushed us to do it because she used to be married and she used to have sex, but then she was divorced and could have it no more. It was safer to be partners with her because she had already had sex so it wasn't like people would look at her differently. Suad had been divorced I believe because she could not have kids. I believe that's what the secret is but I'm not sure.

This was in an eight-floor apartment building and she lived on the seventh floor and my friend lived on the sixth floor so we know her as like a neighbor. She used to babysit for him.

So I was excited about it. She came this day downstairs and always what I hear from stories is that everyone wants to go first. I said I'm going first. This woman and I actually went in my friend's parents' bedroom, and I started kissing her. My friend was waiting outside with all respect. No interrupting or anything. Then I wasn't planning to do it, but she was very horny I guess. And she just grabbed my penis and I was scared and the first feeling, actually it was incredible. Like very warm and very, "Oh my god," and, "Oh!" I have to be honest, I was still scared but I was probably the second person to do that for her after her husband. So I wasn't scared about any disease or anything like that. Then I'll be honest, I didn't want to finish but I couldn't help it! Then my friend started up with her.

My friend asked "How was it?" I said, "I finished so fast. You will too." Then I remember she went to wash and my friend went after me. A week later we were studying together. We were smoking outside on the balcony and Suad came outside and she said, "Do you want to come upstairs?" I said, "All right I will come. Me and my friend." And her face changed and she said, "No, I want just you." I don't know can it be the size? But I know exactly that's what it was. In Egypt it is a little different. We kiss each other and as men we know we're not gay. I can walk in the bathroom while he's taking a shower and use the bathroom in front of him and it's no problem. Yes we trust each other like I'm a man, you're a man, so no problem. But he was like, "Uhhhh...," always hiding. I had a chance to see his penis and it was small. So I figured out why Suad liked me more.

(...and how not to)

All together I was with Suad three times, but we had to stop because our arrangement would look embarrassing and shameful and you can get killed for this. So I can be killed and she can be killed because that's the thing in the religion, the Muslim religion and in that society. If she were still married she could be put in a hall and she can be thrown at with rocks until she dies. And me not being married, I would have 100 slashes on my back as religious punishment.

For husbands or parents, these are her owners. For owners it's totally different. It's like her parents and brothers think, "How can she be a whore? So to claim that her owners to be clear of shame, they can kill her. And they have the right but he will go to jail for that but in a way this is like casual. That's what we do over there.

I PRAY THE LORD MY SOUL TO KEEP
Bjorn, 34

The most interesting aspect of the whole thing was not necessarily the experience in and of itself, but the circumstances in which it happened. Where the act itself was pretty banal, the situation was pretty mind-blowing.

I was raised Roman Catholic and I had a great relationship and a very functional relationship, not the kind of relationship you hear about on the news nowadays, with a Catholic priest. He was a mentor and I used to help him out at the youth center he ran.

When I started coming into my own and becoming an adult and all that sort of stuff, discovering my sexuality, I met a girl who I was totally attracted to. Rachel and I ended up getting together and when we actually did it, I lost my virginity with her in this priest's bed.

So what makes it interesting is, I guess, the irony of it. Roman Catholicism, pre-marital sex, the fact that I had this relationship with a priest, which wasn't suspect by any means. But I lost it in a priest's bed, which was taboo on top of taboo on top of taboo.

I used to work with disadvantaged youth at this facility he ran in northwest Indiana, so I had access to all of the facilities. I had all the keys. He was out of town for about four days so I called Rachel who made the trek from Elgin, Illinois, out to Schererville, Indiana. We hung out and ended up having sex in the only place that was available.

STRANGER IN A STRANGE LAND
Liraz, 33

I grew up in a very religious background – ultra religious; Hassidic, Orthodox Jewish in Brooklyn, New York. Boys and girls were segregated growing up so I really didn't have much contact with boys at all. For this reason I could not have sex in such close proximity to my family; I was way too scared. I was under so much pressure to not have sex until I was married that I just felt I couldn't even be near my family when I did it. The first time I gave myself permission to even think about sex was when I was 23 and I went to study Spanish for a semester abroad in Madrid, Spain.

My family was not happy about me going. The last thing my grandmother said to me before I left was, "Your grandfather is very worried that you're going to have trouble with men." I asked, "What kind of trouble?" She said, "You know... trouble." When I arrived in Madrid I decided that I had to sleep with somebody... anybody.

I was looking around for somebody but every guy who was hitting on me seemed scary, or they just looked too adult for my taste as I was just starting out sexually. I didn't have to like the guy even. My one criteria was that he had to be cute and not scary looking. I didn't want him to look too old for fear I'd be intimidated.

There was a bookstore across the street from where I lived and I remember walking through the door and seeing him at the register. I immediately thought, "That's the guy I'm sleeping with. As long as he's single, that's him."

I went home and told my roommates, I said, "I found the guy I'm going to sleep with." She was like, "Liraz, it does not work that way. Something has to happen. He was to be interested." I was like, "No. It will happen."

Later I went back to the store and I asked him if there was a library nearby. That was my little opening line. He gave me directions to the library but then we just got to talking about random stuff and the next thing you know we were talking for about 10 minutes. That was it; then I left.

A couple of days later I ran into him on the street and he was so nice, like, "Hi," then *kiss-kiss*. You know, like the Spanish do. We talked on the street and he asked me if I wanted to go to a movie so we went out.

At the end of the night we went to this public park where people, straight people, everybody, go to have sex. For gay people it's like a picnic. Straight people who go there to have sex usually know each other already. Gay people, you can watch men pick each other up then disappear into the bushes. Then you see other gay men just watching. It's really weird. Anyway, there's tons of prostitutes, tons of transsexuals. It's a beautiful park and it's shown in this independent Spanish film I can't remember the name of – *All About My Mother*, maybe? Anyway a transsexual goes to this park in the movie and that's where I had sex for the very first time – in that same park.

He started kissing me and he was a good kisser. We went into the bushes to have sex but we didn't have a condom so he got one off of a prostitute and I later found out that he didn't have to pay for it because he had been supplying a lot of the prostitutes with pot so they all knew him.

But he was just adorable, and 17... no stubble on his face so he wasn't scary to me at all – just beautiful, like a little model. But it was really funny because we had to stop midway and he put his pants back on to get a condom and he's running up to all these prostitutes with this big erection.

He was just out of high school and this was funny because he was asking my permission to do every little thing. So at first he was like, "Is it OK I touch you? Is it OK I kiss you?" But then in the middle of sex he was asking about every little thing like, "Is it OK my penis is in your vagina?" I clearly remember him asking me that. I was like, "Yes. I told you you could do everything. Whatever you want to do you can do it." He stopped asking. We had sex and after he finished he took the condom off and he hung it over a branch. After we were done I found out he had a sex education class just before he graduated and they told him he had to ask before doing any kind of sexual act, which explains why he was asking my permission for every little thing. I thought that was funny.

I went home and told my roommate what happened. She didn't believe me so I told her, "Come to the park with me. I bet you the condom is still there." The next day we went to the park and the condom was still hanging on that branch. I had my camera on me so I snapped a picture of it.

NON-MUSLIMS ARE NOT PERMITTED TO ENTER MECCA
Neil, 39

She was Pakistani, a Muslim. Therefore she wasn't supposed to have sex. I'm a Hindu so for me it doesn't make a difference. We do whatever we want. But this Pakistani woman had a boyfriend and everything. She was older, maybe about six years older than me. I met her at some party. I was just playing it off real cool, whatever. She just took me to her place. She told me she had a boyfriend and everything. She really just wanted to do it.

She was the kind of person who did all this bad stuff behind closed doors but then when she was out in public she sort of put on this front. In public she was very, very much an Islamic woman. It was only behind closed doors that she let out her sexuality. She was really good in bed and she was drop-dead gorgeous, could have been a supermodel. It was pretty fascinating for a first sexual experience. I felt it for days afterwards, like arms wrapped around my body. So magical and it was kind of wild to do it with someone who wasn't supposed to.

I remember we got pepperoni pizza. And pepperoni is against the rules of her religion too, so she was cheating on her boyfriend and eating a forbidden food. I think she needed to do everything that was naughty for her culture.

I didn't feel bad. It's not like I was corrupting her, these things were all her doing. I was just young and felt lucky to be along for the ride.

EVANGELICALISM VS. THE REFORMATION
Laura L., 29

I went to private school my whole life and in high school, after two years of dating we finally decided to have sex. So my boyfriend and I went to my parents' house while they were gone and we had sex, nothing big – basic, preacher style sex. And as soon as we were done he got off the bed, got on his knees, and prayed to God to forgive us.

He's saying like, "Holy shit, we're sinners," and, "We're going to hell," and, "Dammit, I really screwed up." And I thought, "Well, I love you. You love me. We're gonna get married. Everything's fine." A full two years after that he still had that angst-ridden, God-is-going-to-judge-us thing so we finally broke up.

We were both from religious backgrounds. He was raised, "You're going straight to hell – Church of Christ." I was raised Lutheran. We drink and we're OK and God loves us no matter what and he's like, "Well, I'm Church of Christ and holy shit and we're going to hell. Ahhhh!" It was awful.

We did try to have sex again maybe once more the whole rest of the time we were together. I wanted to have sex and he got really mad and threw me against the wall and had sex with me and said, "That's it. Never again."

> That night, we had sex in a cemetery because it was nearby. But it wasn't until years later that it dawned on me that I also did it as a way to rebel against my staunchly religious grandmother.
>
> *Ralph, 30*
> *Boynton Beach, Florida*

PAGANS
Jerry, 25

Hell of a chick that Valerie D'Arbanville. There was literally a spark the first time we touched. We were outside walking to class, I went to hold her hand and there was a shock, it was electrical. Yeah, we had good chemistry.

We did it on a bed that had the posts slanted in to form this pyramid shape above us to channel cosmic energy. This chick's mom was into New Age stuff. It was my first time so I have no idea if it helped anything. The cosmic energy sure didn't help me last long, that's for sure.

(…and how not to)

How to Lose Your Virginity

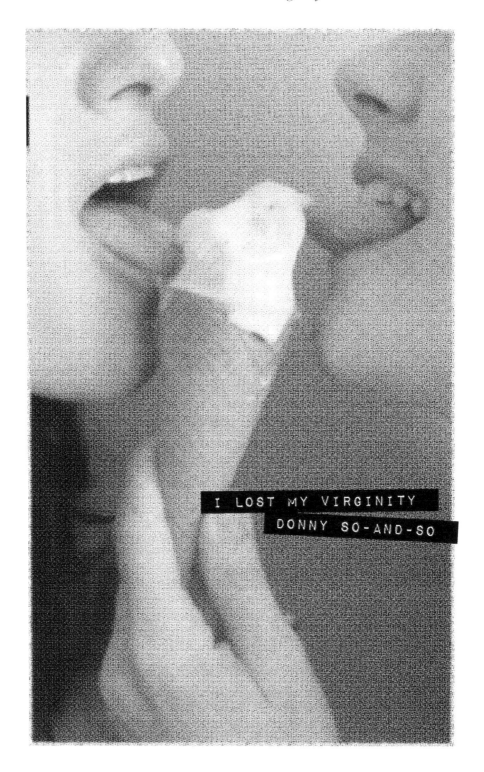

(...and how not to)

"IF I HAD THE CHANCE 2 DO IT ALL AGAIN... I WOULDN'T CHANGE A STROKE..."

14

These have a sense of nostalgia. The stories grouped in this chapter are here not so much for what they are but more for the look in people's eyes as they relived their past. As was indicated to me by Mark, who has the first story in this chapter, "I hadn't thought about that in years."

The chapter title comes from Prince's "Raspberry Beret" and the line that precedes it in the song is, "They say the first time ain't the greatest... But..." for these individuals their first was a declaration, a realization, a discovery that sex is good, sex can be fun.

THE UNDISCOVERED COUNTRY
Mark, 41

I was 16. My folks let me go on this trip with this friend of mine, which was unique for them, but they let it happen. I think my friend was 18 or 19 at the time. He had a Jeep CJ-5 and we cruised around Vermont, New Hampshire. and upstate New York. We were driving back from some wilderness in Vermont, coming into New York, heading to a campground we had seen on the map. It was maybe 11, 12 o'clock at night and there were these two girls hitchhiking on the side of the road. My friend and I just look at each other. So we pick up these girls, the one was tall and skinny the other shorter and stocky. We took them to our primitive campsite which had a bunch of these three-sided buildings that you just threw down your bedroll in. And we wound up having sex with the two girls, one tall and skinny and the other short and stocky.

The trip was a phenomenal trip. Earlier we were camped out on some lake and I caught some trout, gutted 'em and cooked 'em right there and had dinner on the side of the lake. It was such a cathartic trip for a 16-year-old, being out in the wilderness.

This was 1976... 1977, or something like that. And here were these girls on the side of the road. I can't even remember their names, and all they wanted to do was have sex. They were just waiting for someone to drive down the road, pick them up and have sex with them.

It happened pretty much right away, all of us in this tent thing. There was this uncomfortable switch-over moment and it was raw and strange and it wasn't like prom night. The second girl was more fun. She had a sexy attitude, I do remember that. That first time it was like, oh here's this with the first girl then here's that with the second girl. I probably can't do the emotion of the situation justice stating everything so matter of factly, it was actually kind of cool. But then we dropped 'em off at some trailer park and that was that.

Years later I thought back on it, and you know, you have sex with two chicks and you don't know who they are or anything about them, several states away. You don't really think of it when you're 21, or 25, or 29 but when you get to be like 35 you're like, "I don't have any kids, but I wonder if I do."

> I had been masturbating from a young age. And I'm a very sexual person. So it wasn't a surprise to me that it wasn't painful at all. It was just amazing... it was really good. I actually orgasmed, which I guess a lot of girls don't, but I did. And James and I were elated. It just made you want to high five afterwards. You're like, "sweet." You know? We're not virgins anymore. Afterwards we just laid there, grinning like idiots. And from then on it was sex all the time.
>
> Rochelle, 24
> Lyndhurst, Ohio

(...and how not to)

I LOST MY VIRGINITY TO DONNY SO-AND-SO
Michelle, 35

It was with my best friend at the time. We weren't dating or anything, he and I were just really good friends. We were out drinking one night, whooping it up as you're prone to at 19. A girlfriend was driving, designated driver or whatever. We stopped to get cigarettes. Donny knew that I loved strawberries and he walks out with this huge strawberry ice cream cone. He got in the backseat and he kinda like wriggled his eyes at me, so I crawled over the backseat too.

We're sharing an ice cream cone, our friend is driving, and we started making out. I had never kissed him before. The weird part was we had actually got a hotel room the night before because I was too drunk to drive. We slept in the same bed but nothing happened.

So we're making out, we're licking strawberry ice cream. My friend says, "Um, I'm kinda feeling awkward." She was mad because a mutual friend of ours had a crush on him. I tell her to take us to my car. My Chevette was parked facing the beach out where they dock boats in our home town. It starts raining and a Living Colour song was playing on the radio. They were on tour, opening up for the Rolling Stones and had just done an in-store appearance at the Camelot record store I worked at. So I was really into that band at the time.

We finished the ice cream. "Where are we gonna go?" He directed me to a secluded spot and we had sex in my Chevette. July 30th of my 19th year. I always remember the day, I still always kind of celebrate it in a way. Then it happened every day for about the next three weeks. In my car, outside in the park, on the tennis courts.

He drank a lot. He was a troubled guy, a very troubled soul. I think that was part of the attraction 'cause my dad, he's a very troubled guy.

Donny moved but I stayed close to his family.

Two years later I was at a party playing "chandeliers" with this girl; it's a drinking game kind of like quarters. We were drunk at this party playing Chandeliers and this girl flippantly says, "Yeah, well I lost my virginity to Donny so-and-so." And I was like, "Oh my god, me too." She lost hers at 16, I lost mine at 19. We bonded over the fact that we lost our virginity to the same guy and we're still best friends to this day. She's pregnant and I'm her birthing coach because her husband can't handle it.

We both decided we were in love and it was the right thing to do. I wanted it to be special so we got some candles and rose petals. We were in my childhood bedroom and we made love. The whole act from start to finish took probably about 45 minutes to get it right. If one of us messed up, we just took time to figure it out and continue.

Connie, 22
Lakewood, Ohio

CRUSHING ROCKS
Paul, 43

I was working as a clerk in some office. I asked a co-worker out and on the third date she took me down to a quarry on the south shore, 25 miles outside of Boston. She took me there with the intent of having sex with her. I had waited so fucking long. I was in college, that was a long time waiting. I knew before we even went up there that that was the night. It was just a question of where.

We were on the seaside, sitting on a blanket on a big, flat rock. We got a little high, we had some music, like a boom box or whatever. It was a good time. I don't know how much time went by but all of a sudden the tide came in and the rock path we walked out on was gone. We splashed back to shore and where do we go? We climbed on top of a crusher, this big machine that crushes rocks. That's where we did our business. Sweet and lovely.

Awkward? No. Amazing? Yes. I remember having pussy in my face for the first time and then screwing the pussy right after that. What a moment. It was beautiful, it was more than I could have even hoped for. The girl was beautiful, but it was the desire of both of us to do what we did that made it sweet... smooth... ecstasy. Everything about my first time was superb.

RIGHT WHERE I NEEDED TO BE
Rick, 48

It was in Wolfman Jack's basement out in Long Island. At the time I was interning for Wolfman here in New York City. I was helping him and his family one weekend move to California. A number of family members came to help and one of them, his wife's sister, ended up in my bed, in the basement.

It was better than I ever imagined it. It was more relaxed. I performed better than I ever imagined I would have for my first time. It just felt very natural like... this is what men and women are supposed to be doing.

I wouldn't have traded that first experience for anything. She was very sweet, a real southern belle... and for that moment, you know, it really made me feel special and loved and important. She asked me afterwards if it was my first time and I told her, "Yeah." I think she took it as a badge of honor.

She was estranged from her husband at the time and I was prime prey. She was probably in her mid-20s. I was a young, skinny, long-haired, 18-year-old Jewish kid who happened to be helping out Wolfman. Wolfman found out, but there was no repercussions from it. I think he probably would have welcomed me into the family if that ever came to pass. But I never spoke to her again; it was kind of just a one-time thing.

You know when you hear about most people's first experiences they're usually quite awkward... and I felt like... man, this is right where I need to be.

(...and how not to)

IT FEELS LIKE THE FIRST TIME
Emily, 21

What I consider as my loss of virginity is the first time I slept with a woman. It was her first time as well, although we'd both previously had sex with a lot of guys.

I picked her up at a mutual friend's party and then we went to a friend's house who I played softball with. I was a sophomore in college and I had only known that I liked girls for about a month, maybe two. I saw Julie at this party and I thought, "Damn, that girl is hot." I wanted her and the opportunity presented itself.

So yeah, we went back and crashed at my softball friend's place; it was two o'clock in the morning and everybody kind of crashed out. I hadn't been drinking that much, but I started drinking more when we all got there. Julie was pretty drunk and sitting on the counter. I stood over by her and she was leaning over me saying, "What do you want to do?" She got closer and was like, "Can I kiss you?" I was like, "Of course. You're fucking gorgeous." So we kissed and then she goes, "I want to cuddle with you tonight."

With girls it's sometimes like that, pretty innocent. You'll talk and spend the night. We went up to a bedroom but this was different, she was a superfreak. Between the door and the bed she had all my clothes off.

There we are, naked in my friend's roommate's bedroom. First time I ever went down on a girl. You know basically we're just fucking because we're both drunk. My guy friend, Lou, pokes his head in thinking his room is empty and I'm like, "Lou, get out." He was all, "Emily?" because he thought I was in there with another guy. He was like, "I gotta go to work tomorrow." Then Julie told him to leave and he goes, "Julie? Oh, shit. Sorry." He went downstairs and Julie and I had sex for like the next two hours. I did let it slip that it was my first female experience and she hesitated for a second and said, "I'm drunk. I feel bad." I was just like, "Shut up, we're having fun. I'm drunk, too."

Next morning we woke up and Julie walks out of Lou's bedroom and this girl I played softball with and Julie had known for years said to her, "Looks like you got some ass last night." Julie laughed about it and two minutes later I walked out of the room and everyone was like, "Aw, shit." I busted us out in front of the five or six people there but everyone kind of knew I was leaning towards women. That's how I erased the red 'V' for women, the one that mattered.

Next morning was a little funny. We hung out all day. We went to breakfast and watched a movie with a bunch of people. She was getting ready to leave around five o'clock that night and she was like, "I guess I should probably take your number." "Yeah I guess so." That was it, and we've been together about a year.

I still love that woman... that was ah... 16 years ago... she was the love of my life and she still is. I didn't marry her I married someone else. And that's ok.

Bryan, 35
New York, New York

WHAT DOES A KID FROM JERSEY SHOW A WOMAN FROM BOSTON?
Max R, 36

MAX R: I was in high school. I guess she was like 22, 23.

SW: How did you meet this college-aged girl?

MR: I went to a music school, a summer session for high school kids and she saw me. She was pretty aggressive. We hung out a little bit. I think I was too busy. I think the fact that I didn't like girls at all, that I just liked playing music had a big effect on her. So she kept pursuing me to the point where she had to get pretty aggressive or I wouldn't even notice her. And then... I didn't have sex with her when I first met her but she came down and visited me... where I was living.

SW: How far?

MR: I was living in New Jersey and the school was in Boston.

SW: Berklee School of Music?

MR: Yeah, Berklee, of course. So we headed down and one time she came down and visited me from Boston. The bad thing and the most awkward part about it really was that my mom was in the next room. That kept on weighing on my brain a little bit.

SW: She obviously knew some college chick from Boston was there.

MR: Yeah. And that was weird too. Because she had no problem. I'm like, "Mom can Brenda come and visit?" And she's like, "Yeah." And I'm like, "Really? OK." But my mom is super-liberal and really inattentive as a parent... in terms of like supervision. So she slept over for a long weekend.

SW: Your mom cooked her dinner and stuff?

MR: Yeah, she was totally like, treating her great... even though Brenda was there to de-virginize me. My mom was oblivious to that. So was I.

SW: You and your mother are oblivious people.

MR: Yes. Living in a little cloud. I was stoned but my mom wasn't. So, I don't know what her excuse was. And so there was one day when I stayed home from school, 'cause I was in high school still. We started having sex and I was so scared. I'm like shaking and I lied to her and told her that I did do it once before because I knew it was going to be a bumbling mess and I wanted to at least tell her that I wasn't experienced but I had done it.

    I remember sort of just not knowing what to do and I'm like, "Whoa. I'm gonna put a condom on now." And I'm like, "When do you do that?" When is the right time to be just like, "Pardon me for a moment while I do this thing with this piece of rubber."

SW: Had you seen them get put on like bananas or anything? Sex ed. class?

(…and how not to)

MR: No, I had never had that experience.

SW: Had you taken the time preemptively to read the directions?

MR: I may have practiced putting one on but I don't remember. And it didn't matter because I wasn't even… I couldn't stop shaking really. It was so much expectation here of my manhood being on the line.
    So… we did it and I'm sure it was horrible because she was questioning me afterwards like, "You said you did it once with that girl once before?"

SW: She was asking you names, details.

MR: Right, so then I threw in that I was drunk the first time. Therefore I was even less responsible for what happened. But I remember as I'm fucking her I was thinking I should have been, at the time, in Earth Science class. That's all I could think about, I'm like, "Earth Science or doing this real cool girl."

SW: What did you miss?

MR: A test. And then I remember after she went home I called my friend and I'm like, "Dude, remember during Earth Science when you were in Earth Science and I wasn't there?" He was like, "Yeah." I was like, "I was getting a blowjob. And I was thinking of you sitting in Earth Science." And he was like, "Dude, that's awesome." But it was a pretty horrible experience. It wasn't the greatest. It was good and bad, you know. It was a mixture of lots of emotions. My mom in proximity wasn't good. That was bad. The whole mom and sex thing was bad.

SW: She was a stay-at-home mom?

MR: No, she was just home that day. Maybe she was trying to keep me from having sex with this girl. I don't know. I think that was it. The rest was… Brenda still liked me afterwards and really wanted to continue but… I felt I kind of didn't really like her that much. She was also *so* into me that I was like, "Oh, no challenge here." I learned that one early on.

SW: Did you end up going to that school?

MR: No. I had no intention of going there, it was just for the summer. It was too stuffy and weird. And also there was another girl there that was doing the same thing to me. And I was like, "These girls here are crazy. I don't want to go up there." And then after that I really didn't have a girlfriend for a couple years 'cause I just, I was so into music. Girls were such a distraction.

SW: And were girls at the music school you went to crazy as well?

MR: Um… there were like no girls in the school I went to.

SW: Anything else?

MR: I'd like to say in closing that I look back on it fondly. I think it was really fun and I'm glad that she took the time to make me have sex with her. I'd like to thank her.

SW: Just that once.

MR: Yeah 'cause she came down another time; no we did it another time she came down but she totally went schizo that time. And then we ended it. I sent her packing.

SW: What does a high school guy from Jersey show a college girl from Boston?

MR: Charm, man.

SW: I mean around the town.

MR: Oh. I showed her 7-11. The woods you know where we would stash the beers. The Old Milwaukees under the log. And... oh, and my dad ran a theatre. It was like a cultural theatre. It had jazz and classical and dance and all that shit. So I took her to some of the performances there. And then that was really it, 'cause I couldn't drive. She came over and like... couldn't go anywhere 'cause she took the bus down. And it never occurred to me to let her drive my mom's car.

SW: Mom probably would have let her, too.

MR: She would have. She was letting her do everything else.

MANLY DEEDS, WOMANLY WORDS... MARYLAND!
Monica, 25

I had known my boyfriend for like a million years, since high school. We started dating again in my early 20s. We went to the beach on Assateague Island in Maryland one weekend and camped out with a bunch of our friends.

We were both virgins and we were fooling around out on the beach on a blanket. It was three or four in the morning, there was a full moon. There's wild horses out on Assateague Island so the only other living thing on the beach besides us were random ponies walking by.

We didn't plan to do it. It just came to the point where I was like, "I want it." It just kind of happened. Maybe the environment helped, the beach, him, the wild ponies...

(...and how not to)

UN-CHAPERONED FIELD TRIP
Crystal, 30

I'm from Gainesville, Georgia. Little town an hour northeast of Atlanta. I was 18 and it was with my first boyfriend and while we dated for two years we waited that whole first year. He was very patient.

Dylan had gone off to The Citadel in Charleston, South Carolina. The Citadel is a strange military school. And it was strenuous and rough and has all these crazy initiation things like people beating you up with the flat side of swords. They had this rule where you had to obey officers above you no matter what they said and officers would send the younger guys to places they weren't allowed to be in and then other people would be there, waiting to administer corporal punishment. It was just crazy, like he was off at war or something. He could only talk on the phone like five minutes once a week so we wrote these letters back and forth the whole time he was gone. And then I decided, OK, I would. So I wrote him a letter and said I was ready, which I'm sure turned into a bragging point him being at an all-guy's school.

My economics teacher lived in my neighborhood and I had known him my whole life. He knew that Dylan was away, so he offered, "If you ever want to visit Charleston, let me know. I have a condo in Kiawah." I was like, "OK, I'll go this weekend," and he gave me the keys. Economics was my last class of the day so he let me out early and I drove down to Charleston with Dylan's best friend and his girlfriend. My parents were OK with it because we had been together for so long. I'm sure they already assumed we were doing it.

We picked Dylan up from school and he looked so different – starved and all muscle, real manly. We went to the condo and I started to chicken out. We had been dating a whole year and I wouldn't do hardly anything but kiss. He couldn't stay out of school overnight so we had to take him back. But we got back to his school late and he would've gotten in trouble. They would've kept him the whole weekend and not let him out again. It was very dramatic. I was crying.

So he said, "I'm not going back," and he went AWOL for the weekend and came back with us to Kiawah where we had sex in my teacher's condo. We had the beach, each other. It was very idyllic. At that age, you don't really think of the significance of things like having sex in your economics teacher's vacation house. I thought it was really funny. But I was terrified thinking about how severe his punishment would be. He got beat up a bit and was given extra duties.

Dylan and I stayed together for another 6 or 7 months. He wanted to get married, I didn't. I went to college and that was it. Years later I told my mom about it.

Related to the loss of virginity, my dad once said, this was probably the closest he ever came in breeching the subject with me, that you can see a difference in people from before and after. Apparently you start to carry yourself very differently afterwards. That's gotta be rough for a dad to see that in his daughter.

TRANSMISSIONS FROM THE SATELLITE HEART
Bruno, 27

I was in a high school rock band. And we were going to do like the "Monsters of Rock" in our high school. Like a "Battle of the Bands." I was the singer and we covered the Flaming Lips song "She Don't Use Jelly." That was like our big closer. We were kind of a cover band. We had a couple originals but that was our big one. And directly due to us doing that song, a week later this super-cool chick, Sara, she was already doing drugs and everything, she had sex with me.

This was a girl who was way beyond me and my friends. Normally she wouldn't even talk to us. But I sang this Flaming Lips song and she liked the Flaming Lips. But we were at this party at my friend Rick's house and she decided that she was going to have sex with me that night. She was also on ecstasy. She came over to me, took action, basically took control of the situation and dragged me into the swimming pool. We were having sex in the pool with everyone up in the balcony above us watching us. I was like, "Yeah, Sara Donahue!" I was all psyched about it because here was a girl who would never talk to me.

Just recently I actually met Wayne Coyne, lead singer for the Flaming Lips, in LA. He was at the premiere of their movie *Christmas on Mars*. I talked to him and I told him that story. I said, "It was because of you I lost my virginity with this really hot chick." He gave me a pat on the back and he was like, "Nice, man. Glad to be a part of it."

SAVIOR OF THE UNIVERSE
Niles, 40

I grew up in Sydney, Australia. There was this boy at my school. I liked him and wanted to try sex but he was like, "No. You're just going to make me say "yes" and then you're going to make fun of me at school," because I was a jock and he was the gay boy at school who everyone picked on.

We both liked music. That was our connection. So we used to go on friend dates to see like Cheap Trick, or The Knack or whomever. Then I'd drag him to punk clubs to see The Ramones. He used to cry because that the punk shows were so loud. He was more of a disco boy.

One night we went and saw the movie *Flash Gordon*. Kind of a homoerotic movie. I thought it was horrible but I could see it was working on him. In the movie, Flash Gordon was the quarterback for an American football team and I played rugby which, I guess, got him excited. I can credit that movie and the music of Queen with getting me laid at 14. Rather young but I was pushy and he was cute, so it had to happen. We went back to his place and had sex in the shower. We dated for a long time after that.

(...and how not to)

THE WAY TO A MAN'S HEART
Sandra, 29

I lived with my mom and my step dad in a country town called Rock Bank. It's a suburb of Melbourne, Australia of about 1,000 people.

Brent was going to university and boarding with the family next door and my mom really wanted me to date him. She found out he was sick and like the good Italian woman she is, made a bowl of soup for me to take to him.

I went next door with the soup and I asked for an encyclopedia starting with S. I made that up on the spot because borrowing the book gave me an excuse to go back there later and return it. I was just, "Hi, this is some soup and I need encyclopedia S. Yeah, because I'm looking up sea lions for a project and... and I know that you've got encyclopedias and I don't have any." He would take my virginity six months later.

My mother always told me, "If you're gonna have sex I'd rather you have it under my roof. I don't want you having it in the gutter somewhere, or in a hotel room, or in a car." If I was going to have it she wanted me to be in a safe place, somewhere where I felt comfortable. That place ended up being my bedroom one night at about one o'clock in the morning.

It bloody hurt. I obviously had masturbated before but I had never actually put anything that big up that section of my body, and fingers can only do so much. But once you get started, you can't stop. Once I got past the whole first experience, I wasn't just having sex, I was making love.

Then we were having sex all over: my house, the neighbor's house. Mom finally caught on. One morning getting ready for school I had just gotten out of the shower and she says to me, "Your boobs have gotten really big." I was like, "Oh, have they? I hadn't even noticed." She said, "No? They've gotten bigger in the last few months. They only get bigger when they're fondled too much." And I was like, "Oh..." She looked at me and asked, "Have you been having sex?" And I said, "Yes." "Well... as long as you're doing it safely. Just promise you won't do it in my bed." I never broke that covenant and I had already gone on the contraceptive pill so it was safe.

I ended up marrying the man with whom I had my first sexual experience. We're divorced now, but we were together for 11 years. I never appreciated anyone else, so over time, you have no one to compare it to. The whole love part of what we had turned into more of a love between siblings than a husband and wife. But I still remember the first time fondly.

> She had the nicest tits, the greatest tits in the world. I still have naked pictures of her.
>
> *Stu, 28*
> *Burlington, Vermont*

HER SON WOULD HAVE BEEN 16 THAT YEAR
Jack D, 40

SHAWN WICKENS: How did you know her?

JACK D: She was a neighbor and she lived across the street, a hippie from Long Beach, California. I was 15 and she was 42. You are going to love this one. This will be a highlight, will I get a centerfold on this?

SW: Maybe.

JD: It's gonna be a phat one.

SW: Did she have kids or anything?

JD: She had two children. She was born in 1938. And... one of her children went down with her husband in a Cessna in 1975. So she lost her husband and an 11-year-old child in a plane crash, which left her daughter who was born in '57. So obviously they bonded and melded and tried to lick their wounds and got through it. But she was a very cool hippie chick. And my teacher, so to speak.

SW: How did it end up happening?

JD: She was a hippie chick, a hippie freak. Nice lady. Bong hits. Extremely intelligent... I was a naïve 15-year-old, a hippie kid. I grew up here in North Beach. I was a renegade and we just hung out and stuff but she was a free-minded person and stuff.

SW: You had hung out for awhile before this actually happened?

JD: Oh, of course, yeah, months. She was my neighbor, she lived across the street and it had to be a dead secret you understand. I didn't know it was going to go in that direction, but when the day finally came it was one of the most wonderful days in my life. And let me add that I was a geek boy as a kid so I had never even been with a girl before.

So, nice way to break the ice with a lovely 42-year-old hippie chick. I never made out with a girl so you know in grade school you're either one that gets it or one that doesn't. And if you are not, you don't really care because you know you're a geek anyway and it's irrelevant to you. And so there were no big dances, no nothing, you know? You just... eventually everybody's going to lose their virginity. It's got to happen between 10 and 17 (laughs)... those two ages. So I was 15. A very naïve 15, sexually... obviously because I'd never kissed a woman.

SW: What happened that day?

JD: The day... for your specifics... we turned the lights down and pulled out the bong and did a bong hit and she put on Pink Floyd and it was just like, you know the usual.

SW: In the basement or in the living room?

(...and how not to)

JD: No. In the living room. Right there in her house, you know. I mean... we'd known each other for three months. So this whole thing built up over three months to the culmination of the... you know... "thing." We were just smoking and I believe I approached her and I just went and got closer and it was wonderful because... I just got closer and started doing a massage. That was my thing. 'Cause I didn't know what to do... having not done anything before. Facial contact and just sort of this innocent, not knowing what to do and the vibe was there and she was there to accept it and... she took it from there. Not aggressively, by the way. Very, very tenderly and lovely and it was wonderful.

When one doesn't really know what one is doing one sort of lays back and lets the ol' master... I had no idea what I was doing. Needless to say... if you can relax on your back and let her do her thing... "Oh. Oh my god." Dark room and Pink Floyd is playing in the background and... it was wonderful. And again it turned into a whole summer of... very private... encounters.

SW: Was her daughter around?

JD: Her daughter was 23 years old, born in '57. I was 15, I was born in, you know... '64. I had met the daughter, but no. She had no clue and again this was... a very... it was nothing anybody could discuss. It was a very private thing between the two of us, but it was an older lady... stealing a boy's virginity.

SW: Did it continue between you two after that day?

JD: Very much so. It was a summer romance, May 27th I believe. You'll always remember your day if it was a good one. And that was 1979 and it went through the summer. This was a very hectic summer as a 15-year-old. The punk rock scene was going on here in San Francisco and I was running around like a wild child. I was a latchkey kid so... doing lots of drugs, very careless... very immature. Very, you know, not bad but just having a good time and obviously the age gap between us... the woman you know she was very much like a mother, very maternal.

It came to a point, I guess I realized after about a month into it I was very self-conscious when I was around her outside, around the neighborhood, for obvious reasons, 'cause it was an older adult. The whole situation, it had to be something that was very...

SW: Secretive; hush, hush.

JD: Well, sure, think about it... Anyway it went on through the summer and I guess as things advanced... I was having trouble dealing with it. So that was that and I guess it ended around October or so... what I did was I just basically... stopped...

SW: Stopped going by?

JD: She would keep calling and calling. I couldn't deal with this. And at the time my mother's drunk boyfriend was at home... like Jack Kerouac, dysfunctional family... he was dying of cancer. I was a freshman in high school and he was literally dying of cancer in my house, I mean chemotherapy and all that stuff so I was obviously going through what I understand now to be a lot of different traumas.

And obviously with the age difference... I couldn't take it, and I was a renegade. I was running around doing a lots of other things so...you know the combination of all those things when you're 15. But sexually that's the best parachute drop out of a bomber I ever could ever hope for. She was a love, and we were friends for years. And she passed away from cancer just a few years ago. Very quickly. It was really sad to me because I'll always love her, very much. Just, I mean... a mother... a very, very caring person. That was extremely sensitive in a maternal sense to what we were doing. It wasn't a rape. So it was wonderful. And I'm glad you asked.

> It just so happened that the hills around here in town, they were on fire. And my whole room was like ablaze orange. And we had been talking about it for a couple weeks, seemed like the right time. It was beautiful because the whole world was on fire at that moment.
>
> *Dion, 30*
> *Sparks, Nevada*

CHEERLEADER FANTASY
Whitney, 23

It was with my high school boyfriend, Brett. He and I had waited to have sex for forever and when we finally did it, we did it in my house on the living room sofa with my parents asleep upstairs. What I think was beautiful or poignant about it was that it was right after a football game and I was a cheerleader. So it was that wonderful, classic scene of a cheerleader with her skirt up, welcoming her boyfriend. The parents are upstairs sleeping with the door open, completely oblivious to their daughter getting deflowered.

My first time was really quite enjoyable in every way. It didn't hurt, I think because I had waited and I felt really strongly about the person. And what a fantasy for a lot of guys to have the cheerleader outfit. My parents weren't woken up by the sex or by his yelling "I love you" up to my bedroom from his car in the driveway.

(...and how not to)

CENTER STAGE
Alan, 48

I grew up in show business. I was a child actor. By the time I was a teenager I had already been doing shows on Broadway.

I hadn't lost it yet and frankly I don't like that word, "lost." No, I didn't lose something, I gained something. So I grew up around sensuality, sexuality. I was a very driven kid through my circumstances of having a career and performing so I wasn't about going out and getting it on.

When I was turning 17 I took a job in Nashville as a backup singer for all these famous country singers at the new Opry House, people like Linda Ronstadt, Merle Haggard, or whoever was there. I was doing really well and I was having a really good time. As you probably know you always have your backstage entrance for the talent so every time I would go in, there'd be a huge limo there. A girl, this young singer, would get out of the limo and immediately get rushed away. I think this was four or five months before my 17th birthday. She was coming up on 16. And we were always supposed to stay away from this particular limo, even though we were talent also. I'm going in this private entrance and this limo pulls up everyday and I see this figure, this very young but attractive figure, get ushered inside. She's in sunglasses, incognito that kind of crap. But I already dealt with that on Broadway. It was nothing new to me. It happened that I started singing backup for this particular artist, this young girl, who I won't name.

I was singing backup for her, me and five other guys, but her and I had this attraction. Then it was a passive courtship. We were forbidden any interpersonal contact with her but we were on the same stage every day. I'm doing my thing, she's doing her thing. She was shrouded around by people so there was no way to even say, "Hello." She was rushed in with men in black and did her thing and then she's rushed off by bodyguards. Believe me, her people hovered. I'd just go to the backlot get in my car and go home. But something started to happen on stage where, as a backup singer, I started to pick up more than I was supposed to do. I started to feel her vibe. The way she would move.

A lot of people got cut because they wouldn't be in sync with her. But I could keep up. On stage, in rehearsals, and sometimes during actual performances, she started seeing that I could pick up the vibe and she would go off in these kind of improvised vocalizations. She would throw some body movement or a sensual rhythm my way. The other guys would be going, "What? Huh? What's going on?" So we started to get close on stage when the bodyguards weren't around. It was our only opportunity to connect.

But it was very, very sensual. And when you're performing with someone you have to kind of get into the person that you're backing up. You have to really get into their head, get in their body and really understand what's going on. So that was all developing and then we would sneak times to talk. We took more time on stage to check in with one another. We'd steal off to this empty sound stage to converse every chance we'd get. We established that as the way we could communicate behind all the producers' backs, her bodyguards, everyone watching her.

We had been rehearsing for three months and performances had been on their feet for one month when we all found out we were going to tape a television special with, oh, I don't know, like Sandy Duncan and Dennis Weaver and whoever.

We're at the after-party, I had something to drink, things are pretty relaxed. My agent isn't watching me and her people aren't watching her. I went to the men's room and I was going to the bathroom in the urinal. I heard somebody enter and the lights went out. I think, "OK what is really going on here? Who's in here with me?" This is show business, it could be anyone. I'm standing in front of a urinal and this person started fondling me. Then I smelled a familiar scent, it was her. We knew a back way to our soundstage.

This was my first time and she was younger than me and she guided me, she had a lot of chutzpah. We made love and that was my first time and we arranged it with the bodyguards, my agent, my producer that we could spend time together.

After I lost my virginity, or after we gained that from one another rather, it was difficult to hide our emotions. But it was less difficult than wanting to be together and not being able to. We had our secrets and we had our fun. We had our people who kept them for us, the one bodyguard who would slip her through to my place. It was very sweet, very fun, and very titillating.

SLEEPAWAY CAMP
Eileen, 21

This happened in Arlington, Virginia. I was 17 and I entered a summer program called Governor's School for the Arts. It was a month-long program paid for by the state where we took a lot of classes and went to lectures. I was there for visual arts studies and this guy I met was there for humanities.

The first time I ever met Tommy he was sitting on a couch and I was laying sort of underneath him on the floor with one of my friends. She and I were goofing off, being giddy girls and I accidentally licked his leg. I was pantomiming like I was going to lick his leg, but I overshot it and actually did lick his leg.

My friend was making fun of me: "Oooh... you guys are smitten. Oh." And I was like, "No. It was just a mistake." I still hadn't seen the guy at that point but then I sat up and we looked at each other and shook hands and shared a "Hey, that was a little weird." After I noticed him I did get really sort of interested in him. In the long run it turned out to be an effective way to meet someone.

That was halfway through the program so there were two weeks left. We dated for awhile long distance, this was in July, and then I went to visit him in mid-August and stayed at his parents' house for a week. We were very awkward around each other. We hadn't seen each other for about a month and we were trying to catch up, but when we kissed it felt strange because his parents were always around and they were very, very strict. We could never schedule any makeout time or anything.

Towards the end of my stay a bunch of us from the program were having a bit of a reunion and went to see *Rocky Horror Picture Show*, all dressed up and everything. I didn't know any of the characters or anything because it just so happens I was also a Rocky Horror "virgin", so my costume was pretty generic, lots of black and fishnet.

(...and how not to)

After the movie we all headed back to another guy we all knew from the program, Jamie, to his house where all of us were staying for the night. We were all drinking or smoking or sort of lounging around. I had to leave the next morning and my dad was picking me up at eight in the morning to go spend a month in New England with my grandmother.

So me and Tommy were hanging out on the porch swing, our last night together. Everyone else went inside to get stoned in Jamie's room, which had a window overlooking the porch. Tommy and I were on the porch swing making out and slowly we start losing clothes. People were laughing at us through the window and at one point he threw my bra at them.

He asked me, "You're on the pill right?" which was responsible of him. I think that was his way of opening up a discussion on sex. He could tell something was wrong and I did have a really bad headache and he says, "Well... you know what's good for relieving headaches don't you? The female orgasm." I just started laughing and we started kissing and more clothes came off and that's when I thought, "Oh, he wants to have sex with me. We're gonna have sex. Am I ready? Do I wanna do this?"

I had chances before to sleep with other guys and I always thought I was ready, but none of the previous guys were ready because they were immature assholes. Tommy was different and while we were there on that porch swing I thought back to earlier that day when we left his house. He had picked up some book I was reading and he was like, "Do you want to take this with you?" I thought that was thoughtful how he would notice and mention a thing like that so I thought, "A guy who would do that, yeah I'll have sex with him."

There was lots of fumbling until we actually got it. It was pretty early in the morning and while we were having sex I could see the next door neighbors come home and walk up their steps. I forgot about the headache, but only because the pain went elsewhere, so his method didn't completely work. Oh, and there was a full moon outside. Afterwards we were laying there being kind of quiet and then I was like, "That was my first time." Then he said, "Mine too." I burst out laughing, I didn't know we had both just lost our virginity together. We sat out there for a long time and just talked, it was really nice.

We weren't aware until afterwards that our friends were watching the whole time through the porch window. Our heads were towards the window but I was on my back so couldn't see anything anyway. Tommy could tell, but I doubt he was paying attention to anyone watching. Our other friend Albert, who was gay and had a bit of a crush on my boyfriend, came out and said to him, "Yeah, um... nice butt."

A couple hours later someone else sprayed me down with perfume 'cause she said we "smelled like sex." My dad picked me up and when I got in the car he said I looked real tired. I just said, "Yeah. I didn't get any sleep last night." Then I just pulled out my CDs, put Poe in my CD player, put on my headphones, and listened to their song "Not a Virgin" over and over again.

THE SUMMER OF LOVE
Hazel, 25

William. It's strange, I still think of him whenever I'm going through rough times. I just dreamt about him the other night.

My first love and I started dating when we were 16. We dated for years and I'm still in love with him, but that's a whole other story. I was a really rebellious teenager, not just rebellious against authority, but also my cohorts. Therefore I wasn't particularly interested in partying the typical way high schoolers are supposed to. My boyfriend was the same way. We were kind of punk rock kids who did our own thing, independent from our friends.

This was in Ann Arbor, Michigan, and it was one of the greatest adolescences ever. We had a lot of adventures there. We were really kind of like each other's first sexual explorations or whatever. We dated for a couple years and then we broke up and it was this really horrible epic breakup and we spent a year getting back together and breaking up and getting back together and breaking up. I kind of dated other people in the meantime but nothing serious. I mean, with William and I, we're talking epic first love here. And I always thought it would be right for us to lose our virginity together. It seemed right in a way I can't explain.

We were just a couple weeks apart in age so this was the summer we were both about to turn 19. We were getting up there in age and just had one of those intense reconciliations. We got back together and I remember really clearly, it was the night before he turned 19 and we were about to leave on a freight train hopping and hitchhiking trip.

Although it was incredibly painful and not particularly good, it felt really monumental that we could be together and it was really nice because he was the love of my life. It's kind of funny, I always slept with a nightlight because I was scared of the dark and afterwards he got up to inspect the condom by the nightlight to make sure it hadn't broken. He started freaking out and crying saying, "There's blood." He was worried that I was hurt. It was really intense and I was like, "It's OK." Then we both cried a little bit and just held each other all night long under the glow of the nightlight; a relic of my childhood years. It couldn't have been more poignant.

The train-hopping journey was cut short; it lasted only about a week. I was leaving the country for the rest of the summer so we had to get back in time for me to go overseas. We dated for a little bit more that summer. Then we broke up and I moved away. That all happened six, seven, eight years ago? I don't know. I feel real lucky. No regrets whatsoever. Regrets later on, you know. But I was his first as well and it was very special. We're still in touch every now and then and hopefully we'll get married someday.

(...and how not to)

BEAUTÉ AMÉRICAINE
Lane, 29

When I was in high school, this foreign exchange student moved in down the street from me. I'm from Aurora, Colorado, originally – it's a suburb of Denver. I was a junior in high school and she was a sophomore, or the equivalent thereof, from France. My family knew the host family who invited me over to meet Monique Junot. Monique's father was a fairly prominent French journalist. I was the first American boy she met and we became very close.

The relationship was platonic but there was an intimacy that was undeniable. She made me chocolate cake for my birthday. After her year in America I went to visit her for a month in France. Her family lived in this beautiful neighborhood called Le Larose – *The Lay of Roses*. There was a neighborhood ordinance that everyone had to maintain a rosary in their front and backyards, so it was a neighborhood of rosebushes. There was also a town square with rosebushes and pavilions and a little garden in the center. It was beautiful.

One night I told her that I was pretty sure that I was in love with her and she said in her French accent, "I have something to tell you." "What?" And she said, "I am too shy and I am not sure how you are going to feel about it." I got scared, I said, "Why don't you write it down." I got myself ready for the big rejection. She passed me the paper, I read it, and she had written down that she loved me too.

We were together, upstairs in the loft of her beautiful home, which was her room growing up that had since been turned into a guest room, the room where I was staying. We made out and then we decided, or I decided, or one of us decided... I decided... that we would have sex.

That next day we went to her neighborhood pharmacy where I would not only be purchasing condoms for the first time in my life, but I was ordering them in a different language. She taught me how to ask for condoms in French so she wouldn't have to go inside because the pharmacist knew her dad.

I said, "Bonjour. Une boîte de condoms satisfont." To which he replied, "Grand ou petit?" Large or small. So I said, "Large... actually, I'll get both," because I wasn't sure. Anyway I ordered the condoms and went back to her house. That night we made sweet, sweet, beautiful and yes, very awkward love.

The details of the actual lovemaking are... private, 'cause the sex... that was between her and I. But I will say that this first time happened within the first couple days of my month-long trip. Then I had a hard on for the next three weeks. As far as I know, her parents weren't aware of it. They may have guessed, but we never talked about it.

After heading back to America I felt a sense of loyalty to this woman and turned down or sidestepped other opportunities where sex could have taken place. I tried to remain loyal to her because I was so convinced that we would be married and live our lives together. Thus was the manner in which I was raised, but with Monique and myself it was not meant to be.

BLAM!
Will, 26

I'm from Canarsie, Brooklyn. She was from Brooklyn. I never thought it was going to happen with her, but it did.

We first met at a high school assembly. I saw her from the other side of the room and dipped through the entire crowd looking for her. After making my way through hundreds of people to find her I was too nervous to say shit to her. Later I was in class, her friend was sitting next to me and she said, "Oh, I saw you with my home girl. Yo, you should talk to her. She liked you." I was like, "Oh, shit. That's great." Next time I saw her I wasn't as nervous. We wound up hooking up, smoked some blunts, we hung out a few times.

The time I had sex with her was I was in my room and my boy was in the living room waiting for his girl to take the train and then we were going to pick her up as soon as she got to the train station. In the meantime, me and her were alone in my room, and I couldn't get hard because I was nervous. I was laying in bed with her and I couldn't get hard so basically I gave up. I was so fucking pissed off. I sat down and started watching TV and then after awhile I forgot we were supposed to have sex and I started making out with her again. And then I got mad hard and the second I got hard it was a wrap. She put the condom on me and I'll never forget this – I was laying down and she kind of like swooped down on top of me and grabbed my shit and put it inside of her.

I was like, "Oh, shit I'm inside of a girl." But it was numb. I had this condom on, there was this barrier between us and I couldn't feel anything so it wasn't very pleasurable. We were only doing it for a minute and a half and then my boy pounds on the door and he's all, "Yo, we gotta pick up my girl, she's at the train station." I jumped up and pulled my pants up real quick. She got dressed and we bounced.

We pick up his girl, we're all in the car, and we hang out for the rest of the night. No one said anything about what went down earlier in my room. After the night was over I dropped off my boy and his girl and then it was just me and her again. Before I dropped her off home we were like, "Let's go park somewhere and go finish our business." So we did. She was a Spanish girl with a thin waist, beautiful brown Hershey nipples and hair like Slash from Guns n' Roses. Thick, curly hair and she looked like a model. She had a tattoo in between her tits of a star and like a sun with some bursts of sunrays that shot out squiggling over her tits. It was beautiful.

We finished and after I pulled out I realized I was using the condom I had on from hours and hours before. I still had it on that whole time.

Basically it was a minute and a half the first time and the second time was two and a half hours. You know people exaggerate after years and years, it may have actually been an hour and a half, but the second time was still a very, very long time. It was incredible, I'm talking multiple orgasms. It was my first and she got blammed out.

(...and how not to)

GIRLS LIKE TROUBLE
Naomi, 45

When I was in, I think, eighth grade I came out of the auditorium after lunch and there was this guy, oh my god, this cute guy standing there on the side of the building and I thought, "Where's he from? He's not from our school." He wasn't a student. He was just some high school-aged bad guy hanging out and checking out chicks at the junior high. He had long hair and he was really cute. And I was like, "Oh my god. Who is that?" I just got this feeling of complete lust.

I went out one night with a girlfriend and she fixed me up with some boy. I didn't really like my date, but I planned on kissing him because I figured I needed the practice but then I saw that same bad guy from outside the auditorium at the movie theater. I dropped the guy I was with, and that's when I first officially met Wayne. I could tell he was really into me so I lost the other guy and spent time with Wayne. He was from San Jose, but he had gotten into trouble with drugs so he was staying in some boys' home up where I was from in Sacramento.

So we were dating for awhile and my friend Ashley was dating some other tough guy from the same boys' home and it became this pressure point of like, when you can do it or when should you do it. So there was a night she and I decided we were going to go to the boys' home and sleep with our boyfriends.

We snuck in the window around 11 o'clock and I went into Wayne's room and she went into the other guy's room. There were girls probably sneaking in all the time because that's where all the cute, bad guys lived in the neighborhood.

I was in Wayne's room and it was scary in there because there were other guys in the room. We were on the floor in the corner and I was thinking, "Oh my god, there's other people in these beds. I can't believe I'm doing this." But I was so enamored with him. I was so in love with him that I wanted to do it so bad in spite of the less-than-perfect setting.

My girlfriend and I both did it for the first time, we snuck back out the window, got back on our bicycles and pedaled for home. Then it was the weirdest thing. We were riding our bikes, it was about midnight and we crossed paths with this guy we knew from junior high, some big meathead dude who was riding around on his bike all drunk and he was like, "What are you girls doing out this way?" I said, "Oh my god, Ashley don't talk to him. Pedal faster." But she blurts out, "We were just over at the boys' home." Sure enough he pedaled after us 'cause he's thinking "The boys' home? Sluts. I'm gonna get some too." He started coming after us and next thing you know it was a big race to get home and away from this meathead. We're beating up on our bikes, going really fast trying to ditch him and luckily he was drunk so he couldn't keep up.

The next morning there was all this talk about how Ashley had bled on her boyfriend's sheets and Wayne was wondering why I didn't have any blood. And I'm like, "Well I really already lost my virginity shoving a tampon up there." That's really how I lost my virginity. It was a weird, romantic story, but he eventually had to go back to San Jose and we were just kids.

He was into drugs, he used to smoke angel dust and PCP and I didn't know this until I actually went to visit him one time. I lied to my mom and I said I was going on a field trip to San Jose. Me and Ashley again, she was my partner in crime, she went with me. We went to visit him in San Jose and I got to see what his life was like, where he actually lived. He lived with these two grandmas, like a foster home, and he was just a drug guy, I mean he like rolled this joint and I just thought it was a regular joint so I smoked some of it. Next thing you know I felt like I was 2 ft. tall, then I felt big, then I felt like I shrunk again. The stuff was wacko and laced with something and I realized that he really had a drug problem. After that I was like, "Yeah, I don't know if I'm crazy about Wayne.

But my first time was with somebody I really did love and I do still think of him sometimes to this day and wonder what ever happened to him, because we did have a relationship. We were even talking about getting married. Years later after I did marry and had a couple of kids I got this love letter from him, like a, "You were the best I ever had. Best girlfriend I ever had," type of letter. And I still have it.

> It was good. After that I ran back up to the school for basketball practice... and I dunked that day. I had tried before but I kept on kinda getting hung on the rim. But that day I dunked on my first attempt. On my first try after the experience. I just focused on it and did it.
>
> More dunks. Way more ladies after that.
>
> Warner, 27
Mobile, Alabama

(…and how not to)

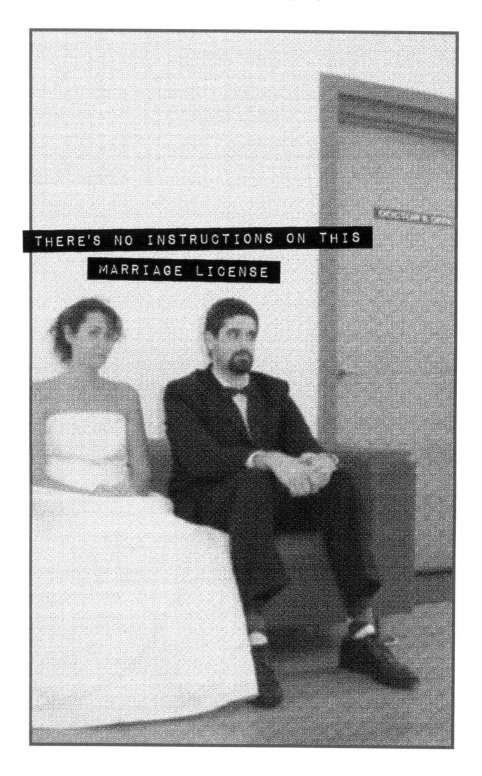

(...and how not to)

"GOING TO THE CHAPEL AND WE'RE GOING TO GET MARRIED"

15

The small number of people I met who waited for marriage I feel speaks not only on the shift of our times, but points to a generational change as well. Very few older people I spoke with who had waited for marriage were willing to openly share their story, as opposed to the hundreds of people closer to my age who didn't blink when asked about their sexual pasts by a complete stranger.

Of the married people I spoke with who did not lose their virginity to their spouse, some shared while their unamused significant other looked on, arms folded. Many of these couples were even unaware of how one another lost their virginity.

These next three stories were the only people I encountered in my travels who saved it for the honeymoon, and in one case, had to wait until some time after.

ORTHODOX
Chaim, 26

Losing your virginity is a very special thing. It is a time when two physical people combine, unite and become one special person. Therefore, we waited until the night of our wedding to create this special bond between us.

We got married a month ago in Montreal, the city she is from. Her brother introduced us. Part of the celebration, the newly married couple goes into a room to be alone together. But the sex doesn't happen there and it doesn't happen five minutes after you leave the wedding.

The Jewish community as a whole, I cannot tell you, but I would say that 90 to 95 percent of the religious community waits until marriage. Most of my friends, I'd say 97 out of 100 have actually waited.

I think older people in the Jewish community give a better example. We look at sex as a special, emotional union between a man and a woman. It's not an animalistic urge to get over with. It's a special time in our lives, a special time for a man and a woman on an emotional level. It has nothing to do necessarily with religion.

It's not the popular opinion but in the Jewish community, most of the time you'll find that families are more open about sex. They do discuss it with the kids and they do explain to them the need to wait until marriage, how special it is if you wait. That has a big impact on the child. My parents explained this to me and it made sense. It's just about parents having an open dialogue, an open relationship with their kids, not to instill fear in their kids.

TALK DIRTY TO ME
Carol, 58

1967, I was 19. He was my high school sweetheart and everything, going together since the ninth grade. Back in the '60s it was just natural to wait until the wedding night. We got married on a Saturday and my husband was registered to start college in Albuquerque on Monday so we really didn't have time for a proper honeymoon. Late Saturday night we were on the road headed for our first real apartment a few blocks away from the college campus. It was raining real bad, the roads were starting to flood so we pulled over and got a room.

The bathroom window was busted out. We had two double beds because it was the last room in the hotel. After I lost my virginity we changed beds. My husband asked me, "Well, how was it?" I said, "It was like 7-Up." "What do you mean?" I said, "Because it was kind of wet and wild."

(...and how not to)

THERE'S NO INSTRUCTIONS ON THIS MARRIAGE LICENSE
Giancarlo, 59

My wife and I waited until we were married and we couldn't have sex on the honeymoon night because, well, my wife was too small. She had to be stretched. We had to wait three or four weeks.

The next day, after we tried, she called her sister because she thought maybe there was a problem. But her sister suggested she talk to her gynecologist. Then after our honeymoon in the Poconos, she called her doctor and made an appointment. After he examined her, after she... it was a female doctor, she examined her and then had a talk with us about sexual intercourse in case we have been doing something wrong. But we weren't.

My wife thought that I was a saint for waiting so long after the honeymoon. I waited that long, might as well wait a couple more weeks. But it was still tough the first time. It wasn't easy because of the situation. She had to be stretched and the doctor showed me what I had to do (makes gesture) ...two fingers and... (spread).

That's what we had to do. We joked that maybe I was too big for her.

> With this ring, I thee wed, and with it, I bestow upon thee all the treasures of my mind, heart, and hands.
>
> *- Traditional Wedding Vows*

How to Lose Your Virginity

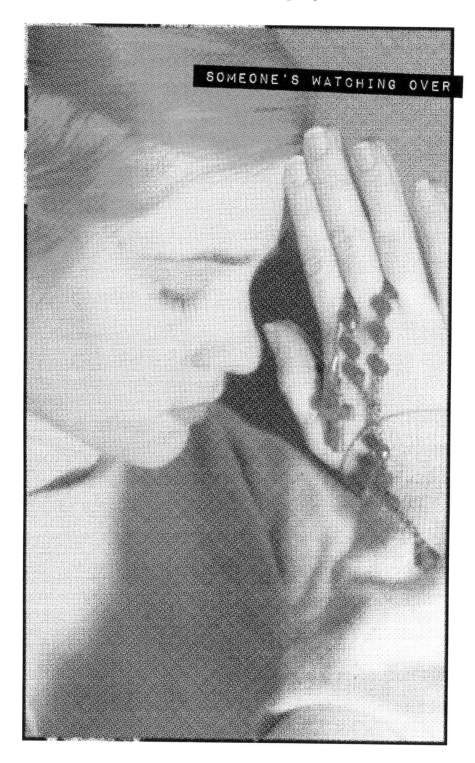

(...and how not to)

"I NEVER DID IT!"

16

Along the same lines as the waited-until-marriage stories, it was similarly difficult to find those who were still waiting. I can recall being a virgin and while I never had a real huge problem with it, it was something I didn't like to admit to friends. As a secret, I could live with it. It was when others found out that I felt ashamed. So I can empathize with Darren, whom I met on his 22nd birthday while he was wrestling with his own choice to abstain.

In one instance I spoke to a college student who, not for a lack of trying, had yet to lose it because of his aversion to physical contact. At the end of the interview when I realized my faulty tape recorder only recorded a small portion of the interview, I asked if he wouldn't mind recording it again and as relief washed over his face, he politely declined and rushed away. I'm sure there were others I asked along the way who also declined to comment out of embarrassment.

Later, while road tripping through Western Texas (perhaps geographic factors were at play or perhaps it was merely coincidence), in one evening I met three gentlemen, all in their 40s who declined doing interviews because they said they were still virgins and were too embarrassed to talk about it. I pressed each one of them, "Really? That's a story that I'd really be interested in hearing." Each reaffirmed their virgin status but again refused.

Unlike other major life milestones, getting a driver's license, graduation, becoming of legal drinking age, losing your "v-card" can seem beyond your control... at times unattainable. So, for all those virgins out there, you are not alone.

SOMEONE'S WATCHING OVER
Hailey, 24

It was a promise I made to my grandmother. Well it was a combination of things. It was a promise I made to my grandmother when she was dying. And I just kind of said it and didn't mean to but I never had a boyfriend before my current boyfriend where I really wanted to. Like, with all my other boyfriends, I felt really dirty. Previous boyfriends would touch me and I seriously would be sick for a week. Before Liam nobody even went "south of the border."

My family's Catholic but it was never like a Catholic guilt thing. It's just a whole slew of things. I had a hard time when my father died when I was 11. I had a hard time with the "He's always watching" thoughts that family would feed me to make me feel better. But it probably ended up messing with my head more than it helped. I made the promise to my grandmother when I was 19, only a couple years ago. My grandmother just said, "I want you to stay... until you're married." It was something I agreed to in passing.

But actually there's a whole other reason now. Liam and I broke up last October. And before we broke up, I was actually going to do it... because, I loved him. But then we broke up because he cheated on me.

There was an incident, three incidents, one girl. Anyways it's an even bigger deal for me now. Now it's... I just want to be sure. So often I'm like, "Uh, I could just do it." But I have such a bad sense of guilt that, once again, not Catholic, it's just I have a really overdeveloped sense of guilt.

So yeah, that's it. It's a combination of things. It's my father, it was my grandmother, it was my family in general. We never really talked about it, but like... my sisters are all... they've all done it. And I'm pretty sure my cousin has too and she's like 20.

The strange part about it is that nobody believes me. My family all thought I was doing it with Liam the whole time. It's not that I don't want to. Liam thinks I have a lot of issues; pregnancy is another issue. I'm terrified of getting pregnant – terrified. I'm kind of on a path with my career now and I don't want to screw it up by having a baby out of wedlock. I'd be kicked out of my family. So it's a whole slew of different things, least of which is the fact that I don't want to do it.

Sometimes I think I'll regret not doing it. Right after my boyfriend cheated on me I thought if I would've just done it he wouldn't have had to go elsewhere. That's crossed my mind a couple times. Plus I've always wanted to be the good girl.

Sometimes he tries to convince me. He wouldn't be human if he didn't. He wouldn't be a man if he didn't. But it's not even that I need convincing. I want to do it. And sometimes it's the hardest thing I do to not have sex with him. There were times like right after we broke up, I was like, "Huh! I should have done it." But in the same vein if I would have done it I would have felt so guilty. There's times where, I swear to God, I think, "What the fuck am I doing? Why don't I just do this?" That happens a lot. He's just a real sport for putting up with it.

(...and how not to)

TIME TO GRADUATE
Darren, 23

I'm in film school, in my last year. And I'm still a virgin. I've had chances. There were a couple of experiences back in high school where I could have gone through with it. But I haven't. I don't know if it's that I haven't felt ready. I think it was more like I was too scared to actually go through with it. Then in one of the situations we didn't have any kind of protection so that's why it didn't happen that time. But I think the main reason is because I really haven't found anyone that I really want to take that step with.

Twice I almost had sex with girls who I knew had gotten around and I didn't want to be just another guy on someone's list. I wasn't like setting out to make a statement or anything. Nothing prideful or me being up on my horse saying I'm better than anybody or anything like that. It just never seemed right.

It's kind of weird being that today is my 23rd birthday, but it's something I always think about. It makes me feel younger than everyone else in a weird kind of way. I feel more inexperienced to the world.

My older brothers are always telling me that I just need to get it over with and it doesn't really matter who I have my first time with. But I don't really feel that it's something that anyone should just get rid of. I'm aware that by dedicating myself to finding someone special that I'm just pushing it farther and farther away. And I don't know that I feel bad that I'm pushing it farther away. A part of me can't help but feel a little frustrated, but I don't know if that's my own feelings or if it's society dictating those feelings on me. I can't say that yet for sure and I'd like to say it doesn't really affect me, that I don't feel different, but of course I do. It just seems that 23 is kind of an old age to be a virgin these days.

I've talked about this with only a very few girls. There's currently this one girl that I've some interest in. She's 18 so she's feels significantly younger than I am but she's already been with five guys. I want to feel like I'm more mature and older than her, but in that one regard she's totally got the upper hand. It's intimidating, it's definitely intimidating. Ideally I'd like to find someone who is a virgin too but at this point I'm not about to limit myself.

My brothers think I'm being girl-like for doing it this way, but that's the way it has to be. I guess I just have to wait it out because I've already gotten myself into this trend of not settling for just any girl, so I think I'm going to have to stick with that. I may be 30 when it finally happens. Who knows?

FOR REAL THIS TIME
Marius, 28

My wife, my soul mate, had been with five guys before me. We've been together five years and I kid you not, I just popped her cherry three weeks ago. It wasn't in the normal spot. It was up high on the top wall. I fucking nailed it and it said, "*Boom,*" the hymen split. That hymen is fucking smashed.

(see page 18)

DID I OR DIDN'T I
Karen, 18

I'm still a virgin, still flying the 'V'. I told myself that I wanted to wait for somebody I really cared about or at least liked. Technically I guess I did lose my virginity because, well, I knew this guy named Kai, and he was really cool and I thought he was really hot and he said he wanted to fuck me. I was like, "Oh, whatever." I was 17 at the time and he didn't know it.

Anyway he wanted to fuck me and I got really drunk one night and I was like, "Fine let's do it." I went over to his apartment and the two of us are naked. He did penetrate and then he stopped and was like, "I can't do it," because I had told him my morals about how I wanted someone I cared about or loved or whatever. Like I don't care about premarital sex; that's not a big deal. I just wanted somebody that I cared about, but I was drunk and I was like, "I need to lose this shit eventually, right? Let's go for it." So he was in, and he was out, and then, "I can't do it, I can't do it."

And I was like, "Fuck you dude, that's fucking lame. Don't tease me!" So I started sucking him off. That got him excited again and he was getting all manly like, "Oh my god, I totally want to fuck you." And I was like, "Then fuck me!" You know, shit dude. Don't fucking play me. He goes in again and then he was like, "I can't do it, I can't do it." And he pulls out again. All because of something I once said about wanting it to be about love and something intimate.

I only knew the guy for a short period and I think he got freaked out because he figured I would get really attached or whatever. And I'm so fucking sick of guys saying they're afraid I'm going to get attached. Get the fuck over it. All right, I do have a tendency to get attached, but once I realize where we are, you know, it's different. As soon as somebody tells me they just want to be my friend and let's just mess around then I'll be like, "OK." So I guess technically I'm not a virgin, but I don't count it and I'm sure sex feels a lot different than some guy just poking his dick inside. I need to stop telling people that I have these fucking morals and just fuck somebody.

I'm not going to just fuck any bum that comes along. But I've been waiting for so long for love and it doesn't even exist anymore. I talk to people who say they don't date so they can be with whoever they want. Nobody really cares about love anymore. I always had these optimistic ideals about how sex could be about love and intimacy and it just doesn't really exist anymore. Like, barely.

(…and how not to)

How to Lose Your Virginity

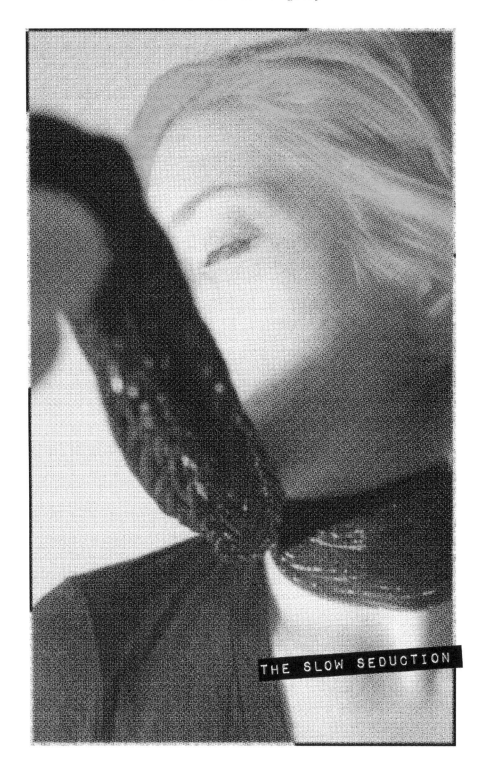

(...and how not to)

"THE OTHER SIDE: TAKING VIRGINITY"

17

After a whole year into the interview collection process I realized I should also be asking people if, subsequent to their own first time, they have taken anyone else's virginity. And the revelation came to me after a man in New York had said his first time was boring but when he "popped some other girl's cherry," that was all the more memorable.

When I began asking this follow-up question, a common response from both men and women was, "I wish." It's a common human need, wanting to be remembered. And it takes a special person to be remembered as the best but far less effort to be remembered as the first; one that just has to show up, albeit before everyone else, to be that coveted "his first" or "her first."

I don't know what's at the root of this drive to be the person to usher someone into their new sexual life. Some of it is well-intentioned, wanting to provide a good experience. Some of it is out of selfishness, a way to assert dominance or power over another person. And perhaps in some cases, it's wanting to relive that first experience as a way to erase one's own lackluster loss of virginity or, as expressed in Madonna's first #1 hit single, "Like a virgin, touched for the very first time," to relive that exciting first moment.

IN MORE WAYS THAN ONE
Holly, 38

After college I lived in San Diego for a summer and I met a younger guy who, like me, was a redhead. A very artistic and interesting guy. I don't know how we met but he was just a really sweet guy and so we started dating.

Everybody thought we were brother and sister because we both had red hair. Somehow I learned the fact he was a virgin so one day we just ended up on his father's boat as it was docked, in the little cabin down below. It was nice because the boat was moving and it was just a really romantic and nice. It was special for him, I'm sure, and I hope that the subsequent times he was on that boat that he thought back on that first time.

He was definitely better than my first time, the guy I did it with my freshman year of college. This San Diego guy just had a lot more sexual energy about him. He was a redhead, after all. And I think the fact that I was older... added some excitement for him.

It wasn't like a big love affair or anything. He didn't fall in love with me after that. Being that he was younger, I thought maybe he would. But he lived in San Diego and I was living in Chicago at the time. I gave him my car when I left, a piece of shit 1979, white Mazda RX-7. I think he got just a few hundred dollars for it from his brother who bought it from him. I said he should use the money to come visit me. I guess that entitled us to one more romp. He had never been out of San Diego his entire life so not only did I devirginize, him but I allowed for him to leave his home turf and visit me in Chicago. I got to devirginize him in more ways than one.

NO PRESSURE
Justin, 23

I just recently went through a breakup and I feel shitty talking about it, but I took her virginity. It was a very serious relationship. We had been friends for a long time and I even felt worse than the time I lost my virginity with someone since there's no way it could have been mutual. I had more experience so at that point it was really just all about her.

She had vaguely entertained the notion of waiting until she got married. I absolutely didn't pressure it, but there was the unavoidable larger arc of it where, obviously I'm interested in sex so invariably that alone is pressure. I offered slowing down and staying friends because if it's not going to be a sexual relationship, 'cause really that's what separates a real relationship from a friendship, then it would have been best to just stay friends. But we ended up deciding and she decided that that's what she wanted. So six months into the relationship I took her virginity. And that feeling of taking something, that irreversible taking... it was 10 times worse than when I lost mine. I was interested in sex and there's no way that that wasn't pressure on her.

Afterwards we were together for about a year before we mutually broke it off. I tried to get back together with her but she refused. During the breakup she even brought up the fact that I took her virginity. I had never felt so guilty.

(...and how not to)

THE SLOW SEDUCTION
Cliff L, 39

CLIFF L: Let me tell you about Veronica. When I was in college I met a beautiful girl named Veronica. She was the prototypical petite chick – 110 lbs., cute, innocent... came in from a little town. And the way that I met her is that I used to work at the little campus radio station at U of L and when women would walk by our window, I'd be obnoxious and wave them into the radio station. I waved Veronica in and when I saw this girl, I really liked her. She had this sort of an innocence, but sort of an energy. You know how sometimes you can look at a woman and can feel that she has a passion but... it's not been realized.

SHAWN WICKENS: Sure.

CL: Yeah, they're absolutely wonderful. They're sort of the librarian types, the academic types. But you can tell that they're just out of control if they get the right stimulus. Well, the way I first met this woman is that I invited her to come in and I told her that we were going to do the balance test. The balance test consisted of her sitting on my knee, and balancing. I had just met this woman seconds before and I balanced her on my knee.

SW: This was on air?

CL: On air. And one of the things I noticed very quickly was that when she balanced on my knee she spread her thighs. It turns out that she had horses growing up. So this was familiar to her. And I knew that I had something special. The thing though was that this girl was just so innocent that I couldn't bring myself to just take advantage of her. And I wasn't really sure that she was the right girl. So what I did basically was I teased this girl sexually for about six months, to make her beg. One evening in particular... I had her in her dorm room and had her stand up next to her bed and I had the silk scarf and she was wearing a little teddy and I rubbed a silk scarf back and forth between her legs and told her to beg for me to please, please, please. And she was just so passionate.

She was one of those girls that just... you know, touching them anywhere, her belly or her thigh, wherever... I got her crying, begging me please to take her. And instead I only put my finger inside her and made her cum, cum, cum again.

Long story, short. All of the other guys really, really wanted this girl. She was the girl that they just had to have, but I couldn't bring myself to take her because she was just too innocent. So I teased her for a long time and at the end I told her we couldn't date because I met a girl who was more sophisticated. I ran into her a year later. Beautiful, and still a virgin.

SW: And still innocent.

CL: I'm in the projection booth at the Red Barn Theater on campus. I was running the film. She came up and I hadn't seen her in a long time. We talked, it was really great. She was wearing a little miniskirt and she came out of nowhere, real strong. She sat on my knee, the same way she had at the radio station. So... we're in the projection booth, it's a year later. I had rejected this girl in relationships because I thought she's just not really emotionally mature enough. And she comes in and she has come for a purpose. She's wearing a little miniskirt...

SW: And she knew that you worked there.

CL: Yeah, yeah. We had spent some time there before. We had made out there. I had teased her there many a time. One of her favorite things was to stand when the theater was darkened... I would stand her looking out over the theater while the lights were out and I would finger her in the dark with the crowd down below.

So she came in and she was wearing a miniskirt and she wasn't wearing anything underneath it. And I hadn't seen this girl in awhile. So she came with a purpose. She came to make me take her. And I felt really, really, really guilty about it because, you know, but... she wanted it so badly she begged for me to please do it.

As she sat there in the chair, I fingered her. And it was so good she just reacted so much. Every tiny little touch of my finger meant so much to her. I took her to my home and we made love for about five hours. You know how when you first, that first tenuous... and there was this amazing sensation when I finally let my penis go inside her she like, gave up everything to me. And somehow when she gave up everything to me I lost all respect for her, and for who she was.

SW: Her innocence was gone.

CL: It made her seem less to me. And she was so sincerely, so sincerely in love with me, but only for the sexuality and the power that it brought to her. It broke my heart. We continued a relationship for a couple of months after that, lots of hot sex that, you know, took it to a higher and higher level, but there was no place for it to go emotionally except the sexuality. And it absolutely broke my heart the day that I had to tell her I didn't want to see her anymore because it was only about the sex.

SW: Right.

CL: And wherever she is today, someday I'll see her again, I'd like her to know that I really, really, really did care about her. And I was only trying to protect her.

SW: Did she, sort of when you told her, did she understand?

CL: No she didn't. She sent me letters and she... started... actually she went kind of nuts. She started exhibiting all sorts of really odd behavior – writing strange notes to herself and leaving them as though I had left them. Went completely off the end. Now... one thing that all really shallow men know is that there's nothing hotter than a psycho chick.

SW: Than a what?

(...and how not to)

CL: A psycho chick. Only truly shallow men can admit this, and I am one – I must be for this story. And the fact that she loved me so much and I didn't love her, it gave me a kind of a power over her that I hated myself for feeling. But I loved the power. In the end, the way that I finally solved it was I invited another girl over and created a situation where the three of us had sex. And it was very clear that she was just another girl being used. I used her horribly sexually. Held her face down and physically used her face and then used the other girl in the same way. And that was how she knew that it really didn't mean anything to me.

SW: Yeah.

CL: I feel so horribly to this day. This is fifteen years ago and I still can barely forgive myself.

SW: I appreciate you sharing your story.

CL: It's nice to let that one go.

(see page 230)

CHECK THAT OFF THE LIST
Katey, 23

I was at an Ohio University Halloween party my freshman year and I met this guy dressed up as Fozzie Bear. I didn't feel like dressing up that year; I was a librarian, I carried a book around.

Steven was very cute, a little outdoorsy guy – kind of emo, kind of indie-rock. I make out with him that night. I don't see him again for eight months, run into him again and we make out again. No big deal.

Three years pass and it's three days before my graduation. I had a list of things to do before graduation: sex in the art building, sex in the library, sex on the 50-yard line, and also to take someone's virginity. I ran into Steven again after all these years and my boyfriend is conveniently out of town so I proceed to take Steven home. He was a 23-year-old virgin. He was saving it for somebody he loved. And I'm just that hot, I convinced him not to wait any longer. I think I might have given him a blowjob, which is really funny 'cause I never give people blowjobs. I had to teach him how to put a condom on. Someone had to, the boy didn't know. It was very entertaining to me.

Every time he was about to cum he thought he had to pee, not understanding what it felt like to cum from sex. In the morning we woke up around 8 o'clock and he's like, "Oh, I'm so glad I lost it to you. You're so amazing." I was like, "Can I say something without it being rude? You need to leave because my boyfriend is coming back to town today." I kick Steven out and I broke up with my boyfriend 12 hours later. During the break-up I told him I slept with somebody because I was mad at him because I found out he had decided he was going to move to California.

But the guy was 23 and waiting and I totally turned him. I call that one my ace of spades V-card.

ANATOMY LESSON
Simon, 31

I was in the seventh grade and I took this girl's virginity. She was the most popular girl in the school and she was in my garage. I wasn't a virgin, she was. I had her in my garage and I promised her it wouldn't hurt. I told her it would be all good. She never had anything up inside of her, but she was the most popular girl in school, so you know I felt I had to tap that.

But I put it in her ass. I had her bent over the workbench and I put it in her ass. She's like, "Oh, it hurts. It hurts." I was like, "It's supposed to feel that way." So I was fucking her in her ass for about 10 or 15 minutes. I was fucking her real hard and I cummed up inside her. She was like, "Ughhh..." She put on her pants and went home.

The funniest thing is I took her virginity twice in one week. A week later she comes over and says she wants to fuck again. I took her to my bed, I'm fucking her in her pussy and she said, "It's in my ass! It's in my ass! Take it out!" I said, "It's supposed to feel that way."

She thought it was in her pussy when it was in her ass, and then she thought it was in her ass when it was in her pussy. I got her all mixed up.

(see page 16)

THE FIRST ONE'S FREE THEN THEY COME BACK FOR MORE
Guillermo, 33

In college, I was a junior and this girl was a freshman and I could tell that she liked me but I would never have sex with her, get intimate with her because I felt like since she was a virgin I would hate to be the one to spoil it for her. I guess her hanging around and me being horny one night led to me making a move on her.

We were the party guys on campus so a lot of underclassmen looked up to us 'cause we always had a party going on. And I happened to leave my door open all the time. And I remember, I came out my shower with a towel on and she happened to be sitting in the room, which was nothing un-normal. It was like that all the time, people just hanging out in the party room. And now that I think about it I probably did her wrong. As I think about it I remember I called four or five other girls to come over to visit me while she was there. I think I lost the towel after the third phone call. And no one else could come over and I kind of looked at her like, "You're here and I'm here... if you won't scream I won't holler." And she didn't leave so I figured it was the right opportunity.

Long story short I ended up hurting her heart. And she ended up becoming one of the biggest freaks on campus. So do I get props for that? Do I get a high five? I would think about five or six other guys on campus owe me a high five for that one there. I made her. That's sad I talk like that. And my dad's a minister. That is so sad.

But it's kind of like the dope dealer thing. If they didn't buy the dope from me they would've bought it from somebody else, I guess... don't make it right though.

(...and how not to)

THE STUDENT BECOMES THE TEACHER
Emil, 36

She worked for me in my restaurant in Maine. We always got along together. She's a beautiful young woman. I was with an older woman for my first time so it's ironic the way this all turned out.

Her and I would always tease each other, play games, and one day it was like, "Why don't you just run away with me..." joking like that. A couple months go by and we continue playing that game, flirting with each other. She has an incredible smile. Then on her birthday, the 12th of July, her parents didn't even say "happy birthday" to her. That upset me. I thought OK I have to do something for her because I really like her, she's a great employee. A friend of mine is a jeweler so I had him make these beautiful earrings for her. No expectations whatsoever except for, she should just be given a gift. You know, how could your parents forget you on your birthday?

It all seemed ironed over but then the next week her parents told her she couldn't stay at their house any longer. I have an apartment above my restaurant so I said, "Lindsey, why don't you stay at my apartment? You can stay there." The next weekend after that, I was over at my own place and she came over because again, her parents kicked her out. So I said, "Come up." I really didn't think anything of it. We watched *Young Guns,* but really didn't watch that much of it whatsoever. We didn't do anything, we were just talking to each other and she's telling me everything about what's going on in her life with school and all of her friends. I just listened to everything she had to say and the movie went by real fast.

I was 35, almost 36. She was 20. At that point in time I just thought of her as a really great friend. Another week goes by and she's at her parents' house and everything sounds fine and then the next weekend she says they're not going to let her stay. During that time there was an oven explosion in my restaurant and so the whole side of my face was burned and my ex-wife couldn't even care less, made no effort to do anything for me... and I could have died.

So I was in the hospital, got morphine and everything. Lindsey and I hung out so another week goes by and once again she can't stay at her parents' place so I let her stay at the apartment. The only thing is, I'm going to be there too since I was laid up from the accident. So we're sleeping together, it's a king-sized bed, plenty of room. She asked me for a massage, which I'm actually in school for massage so the request itself was nothing out of line. I give her a massage and again I had no intention of anything and went to sleep. Then in the middle of the night she woke up and she told me that she always had a crush on me and she wanted to know if I found her attractive and, "Yeah, you're beautiful." We kissed for a while.

It felt a little weird being on the opposite side of the age thing. I told her there was a big difference in experience. And her at 20 I figured she could have only been with a couple of people at that point and whether I should have only been with a couple people well... I'd been with a lot of people. She told me that she'd only slept with one person. I was like, "OK. I understand that, but there's a difference between a high school-aged boy or a college-aged boy and a man who's slept with as many women as I have."

So we didn't do anything, we kissed, we held each other. I told her that I love being with her. We had a great time. The next weekend was my birthday. I turned 36 and she came up to Portland, Maine, with me and we spent the night together. And that was the first time I made love to her and it was obvious to me that the one guy she'd been with really didn't know what he was doing. Later I found out that she really had never slept with anybody. She had gone down on guys, they'd gone down on her but nothing else ever happened.

And we made love for hours and it was enjoyable for her. It was enjoyable for me. I had a wonderful time making love to her. And she is an incredible lover, but the thing is, it took a long time building up to the point where almost a month from the first time we really admitted to having a sexual attraction for one another to the point where we had sex for the first time. I mean we had done a lot more, we had kissed and touched each other, played with each other. There was a lot of intimacy that led up to it which, for me I think, it was like I can give you something as opposed to, you know a 12 or 13-year-old girl having sex with a 13-year-old kid and neither of them knowing what the hell to do. But for my first I had a woman show me exactly what was supposed to happen. So I knew how to show this young woman.

We're still together, but the hardest part now is that I kind of want her to experience other possibilities. That's a difficult position for me to be in. I was the first guy that she ever was with and, oral sex, whatever anyone wants to say, I mean, Bill Clinton was right in that aspect that it's really not sex. It's sex but it's not sex. And for someone like myself who's been around and seen what the whole world of sex has to offer... I can give her me but I can't give what everyone else gave me. It's hard.

(see page 41)

> I would never again want to take someone else's virginity... I felt very terrible about it. It wasn't a good experience for her and I just wanted it to end. It wasn't sexually turning me on because it was hurting someone that I felt for.
> *Randall, 22*
> *Houston, Texas*

(…and how not to)

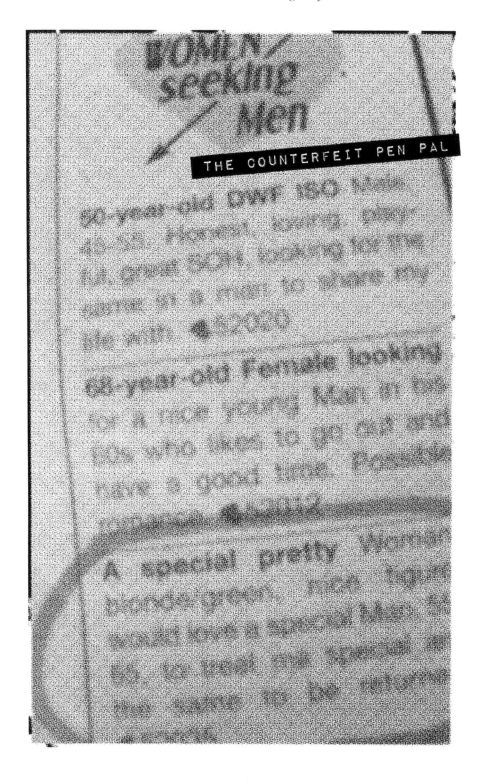

(...and how not to)

"I DID IT MY WAY"

18

Though most of my road trips for this book were solo trips, they felt more purposeful than any other vacation I've taken because I had a specific purpose for traveling instead of sightseeing. And I feel an analogy can be drawn between my positive travel experiences with some people's good first times – if you set out to lose it, just get it over with, that's most likely exactly what it will feel like. But when approached as, "I've given it some thought, this is who I am, and this is how it will best work for me," "I'm finally going to discover the mystery that is sex," "Here it is, the beautiful act that inspires some people to compose songs, write sonnets, paint or sculpt the human form," "I will need training wheels at first but I'm still going to enjoy it," the experience ultimately benefits. Journeys with intent illicit better results than just going through the motions.

How you see it is what you'll get out of it. And while we may not have as much control over when it happens as we may like, we do have control over our attitudes towards it. That not only applies to the first time, but every time.

One aspect of these interviews I didn't expect to find was individuals who knew what they wanted, knew how they wanted it to go down, made a choice and went after it. In these instances, I've found those who defined the parameters of losing their virginity had more positive experiences. Confidence breeds success. Knowledge is power.

ON MY TERMS
Rebecca, 38

We met these guys dragging in Douglass, Kansas, which was where the closest drag strip to Wichita was at the time. I just woke up that day knowing that I was going to do it and it was simply a matter of finding a stranger. Virginity to me was a power thing. I didn't want any of the guys I knew to have that much power over me so a girlfriend and I picked up a couple of guys to have sex with, which nowadays is stupid.

We were all driving around, flirting, hanging out of the cars and we ended up out in the country, right in the middle of an oilfield, right next to the pumps. As those oil pumps were moving, so was I. He was a complete stranger, it was happening there and then because it was my choice. My way, my time. My friend had already lost hers at like 14 or 15.

I never gave in to peer pressure or anything like that, and sex at the time wasn't a big issue to me. I was 18; I was going away to college. It was more of a control thing. Other things were happening at that time that were beyond my control. My parents were getting divorced and their separation was a loss of control, a loss of what I knew. Losing my virginity in this manner was purely a way of controlling what I could – the how, the when, the what and the where... with some guy whose name I do in fact still remember. So it was a very conscious, non-emotional choice. The love thing wasn't important to me. I was watching my parents fall apart so love wasn't the issue. It was control.

There was a lot happening then. I was going away to college and a lot of my friends were staying in a small town, getting married. I didn't want that. I left town and went to college and did it all my way.

ELECTORAL VOTES: 286 TO 251
Lana, 18

I met him at a protest march for peace around a year before I ever started dating him. Then afterwards there was a show put on by the local S.P.A.R. organization, Skinheads and Punks Against Racism, at this American Legion hall right outside Philadelphia. Everyone went to the show after the rally.

I'm not really sure when I decided he was the one because he was tall and very muscular; me – I like lean guys like around 130 lbs. But he's really an awesome guy and had a lot of respectable views on the world and actually followed through with being active on achieving goals and stuff. So I was attracted to the fact that he was ambitious and going to school for what he wanted to do. And punks aren't usually the most ambitious types, but he was a nursing major at Drexel which I thought was productive. We dated for about a month and then came Election Day for the 2004 Presidential Race.

(...and how not to)

I wanted to have something beautiful to look back and remember other then Bush getting reelected – one good memory before everything just went completely downhill. It went down in a Drexel dorm room. I didn't go into it thinking it was going to be amazing or anything. I just wanted it to become a good memory. Aside from it being in a Drexel dorm room, 'cause what's grosser than having sex in a dorm room, it didn't really change the relationship any. I had waited awhile and we had known each other for so long. Then later that day, of course we found out that Bush was reelected. But I still have that nice memory, which is awesome and exactly what I wanted.

It was pretty weird because the whole thing was planned and most people don't plan out that type of thing. He was actually really unsure about whether or not he wanted to be my first because it wasn't *his* first. I told him I was ready and that I wanted to do it on Election Day because we were going to hang out that day anyway and it was just to have one day together as crazy youth before the election. After we finished he asked me if I was OK, then we cuddled and fell asleep.

It was horrible sex. He was a very large black man and it was my first time. I never enjoyed it with him the couple more times we did it and I was afraid I'd never enjoy sex after that. But all in all it was a pretty good experience. I didn't go into it looking for love or for anything magical or life altering. So I guess waiting all that time and going into it with clear knowledge of what I wanted was the right way to do it.

THE COUNTERFEIT PEN PAL
Brenda, 35

I decided to lose my virginity before the legal age which, in England, is 16. On a whim my friend and I bought this youth hostelling magazine so we could flip through the personals section in the back - man desires woman type of thing. Terribly exciting reading for 16-year-old girls.

I thought, "This is the way I can go about it. This magazine is how I'm going to engineer it." And so I found this listing by a bloke in Rumford, which is not very far from where I lived.

I wrote him and we had a very long correspondence for about two or three months. His letters came and I had to quickly rip them out of the envelope and transplant alternate letters that I had written with different handwriting inside, so that my parents didn't realize what was going on. I told mom that this pen pal Neil was really Natalie and that Natalie was in a wheelchair so she couldn't possibly come to visit us. There was a lot of subterfuge going on. And it worked.

So I went to visit Neil or "Natalie" in Rumford who turns out to be a 35-year-old physics teacher. He didn't know I was 15. I lied. I pretended I was 18. Very, very bad of me. But for sure he knew that I was 15 before the dirty deed was done, which I thought was slutty fun.

He did this funny thing... this really bizarre thing like how teenagers play games and throw dice to take their clothes off. And I thought it was really odd for somebody his age to be into that. And so I said, "Let's take our clothes off already. Let's not bother with this bizarre thing." And so we went up to the bedroom and we had sex.

Funny enough I had no idea about orgasms. When I took my knickers off he started rubbing his penis up on the outside of me. I thought it was really fruity. I was very disappointed by the whole thing. I thought that the whole thing was a bit overrated, but I was pleased that it was over and done with and I felt terribly naughty – that thrilled me.

Then he kept writing to me, and I thought, "No, I don't want this anymore," so I wrote to him that my parents had found out about him and that they were going to write to his school if it continued. I can't believe the trauma that must have put him through. But I did what I set out to achieve and I did it in the best way I could think of.

PRACTICE MAKES PERFECT
Carrie, 30

I'd been dating a guy on and off for six months. I lived in Boston and he lived in New York so it wasn't that serious. I was in college and I was dating other people so it didn't really matter.

Then I moved to New York and he and I became much more. I realized, "My God, I'm a virgin. And this guy is like 12 years older than me... what the hell." I didn't want to be inexperienced with him so I went to a party one night and I was like, "OK. Who am I gonna lose my virginity to?" It was so planned, not romantic at all. I literally went to a birthday party thinking, "Got to get this off my list."

So I met this guy and he was so very, very into me. He was really, really, really nice and very doting. We were at a bar in SoHo called Match and there was a sushi bar upstairs. We were eating and I mentioned how I really liked this flower arrangement on the bar and he paid the bartender for it.

So I slept with him. I was sober. I knew what I was doing. I don't know how other women react to the first time, but I was weirded out with it. It did hurt, but it wasn't excruciating.

The next morning he was totally nice but it was kind of sad. He was like, "Let's go to brunch." And I was like, "Actually I'm meeting my boyfriend." I felt really gross about it, but whatever. At least it wasn't with someone completely random; he did know my friends.

I always had this weird thing that I never wanted to sleep with more than 10 people in my whole life, so I don't even count the first guy 'cause it was such a non-event. Maybe a month later I slept with the guy I had been seeing and I was like, "Ohmigod. This is the real thing." We talked about it later on and I was like, "Did you know that I was a virgin?" And he was like, "Of course I did." He thought he took my virginity from me, but he so didn't.

(...and how not to)

CAN'T YOU TAKE ANYTHING SERIOUSLY?
Kate, 21

I was 18. I wasn't the girl who thought it has to be special; I just wanted to trust the guy. Bryce was like 26. I worked with him at Papa John's and I knew I could trust him.

He was dating another girl but he told me he loved her like a sister. He broke up with her so one night we were driving around and I was like, "So..." He asked, "What do you want to do?" I'm like, "Let's have sex." He's like, "Really?" And I say, "OK."

We couldn't go to my house and we couldn't go to his because he had moved out of his ex-girlfriend's place and was temporarily living with a friend and only had a twin-size bed. We stopped by my house and got my little sister's Green Bay Packers blanket; some day I'll tell her what I used it for. We take her blanket and we're searching for a place to go and we find this court in a subdivision that's being built. He and I go into someone's future walk-in closet, lay down and we started going at it.

I'm kind of a jokester. There's this part in the movie *Buffy the Vampire Slayer*, not the TV show, when Buffy is killing the main sidekick of the big, main vampire guy and the sidekick won't die. Buffy is trying to kill him and he's going, *"Ughhhh, Arghhhhh, Uhhhhh,"* and he just wouldn't die. When I was having sex, for some reason that's what entered my head so I'm like laying there and he's like, "This is deep penetration," you know kind of as a joke, so I was like, *"Eeeeeeee, Oooooo, Ughhh,"* every time he went in.

So it was awkward but he was experienced and knew what he was doing and that was a good thing. We finished and we left the condom for the new homeowners or the construction guys to find.

I later on went back to see what the street was named: Homefield Court. It was in a development near a baseball stadium so all of the subdivisions had names that had to do with baseball.

A CAUSE FOR CELEBRATION
Grey, 55

I was always friends with females but I never, ever wanted to have sex with a female. I always considered myself a female. And apparently everybody else in high school did too. They were all assholes to me. Those people were all absolutely awful to me.

I was 18 at Western Kentucky University. I never had any sex with a man but I wanted to. I went into the student union men's room and there was this thing written on the stall door advertising, "If you want a blowjob, meet me here at 7:30." I thought to myself, "Well I don't really know what a blowjob is, but I'll be there."

I waited and this old guy, well he was probably like 27, but in those days 27 seemed old to me. He was 27 and still a student. I think he worked and was going to school part-time. He walked into the men's room at 7:30 and back in 1968 that was about the best a gay man could get in Kentucky.

There was no real conversation except, "You want a blowjob?" "Yeah, that's right." "OK let's go." We got in his car and drove around in the country, which it wasn't too hard to find a secluded place in Bowling Green. He blew me and I came in his mouth and I remember Dusty Springfield was singing "Son of a Preacher Man" on the radio as I was getting my load off. I'll always remember that song playing as I'm shooting my first load.

I thought that I should probably kill myself after that because I had never done anything so sinful. Now, believe me, so much water has gone under that bridge.

He didn't ask me to reciprocate or anything and I never saw him again. Although I did put my mouth on his penis. I really wasn't too sure what in the hell that was all about but he asked me to do it, so I obliged. I didn't suck it and he didn't cum in my mouth.

I'm telling you, that was about the only way you could do it in Kentucky back then. I'm what they once called a "tearoom queen," 'cause if you wanted gay sex you went to a public toilet. There were no gay bars.

But that happened on December 9th, 1968. Of course I remember the date because I was so eager for it. I come down to the pub all the time now on December 9th to celebrate. In fact, I come down to the pub almost every day to celebrate because I'm gay!

EXPLORATION
Cliff, 39

This is the story of a man who in the midst of a great 10-year marriage that produced four wonderful children just got the idea that he'd like to try something new.

We lived in a small college town and there was a local, gay club my wife and I used to frequent because the best dancing and the best dance music is always at the gay clubs. They did drag shows on a regular basis and the queen of the drag queens, the most beautiful girl there was a girl named Chastity. She had beautiful breasts, was very, very feminine all except for her penis and I have to admit that I used to enjoy a little bit of the male attention from her and the rest of the queens.

One night after my wife and I somewhat amicably decided to get divorced, I went down to the gay club with the intention of seeing Chastity and talking about that evening's events. I always tipped well and she had kind of a rapport with me from previous shows my wife and I had attended. I told Chastity that I wasn't going home that night because the marriage was over and she invited me back to her place. She invited to take care of me and she did.

She stayed feminine the whole time and she was wearing this beautiful lingerie and we made out and it was really great. She was so soft. She gave me probably the best blowjob I've ever had in my life. It came to the moment when she took my hand and guided it to her penis, and I call her a woman because that's basically what she was except for that one part. It was incredibly scary, but it was erect and it was beautiful. It was a giant clitoris and it scared the hell out of me. I put a condom on her, put her penis in my mouth and sucked it like it was my wife's breast. It made me feel pretty incredible and set me free.

(see page 217)

(...and how not to)

WITH A SIDE OF BACON
Annie, 27

In British Columbia. Let's see, I was 15 and I was a waitress in a little diner. My boss, the owner, was the guy's mom and he was a dishwasher.

What can I say? We had sex and then we considered ourselves boyfriend / girlfriend. It was in a mobile home, a trailer, three weeks after meeting him.

The evening was planned and in the back of my head I had already been thinking of it as a possibility. I was so ready. I was so curious, I wanted to know that part of living so when he made all the moves I just followed along, went right with it. And yeah, it was good.

Beforehand, I told him that, "OK I've never done this before." He said, "No worries. I'll just take it as far as you want it to go and I'll stop when you want to stop." He was really good that way. Then of course the issue of contraception and birth control came up and we did it responsibly.

Afterwards it felt really cool. Almost like I had passed a threshold and I was now a woman.

I was in a state of euphoria. I felt high. I was high on life. Nothing felt harsh. Everything had this beautiful hue, like looking through rose-colored glasses. The world was good.

I know a lot of girls have had bad first experiences but I had a good guy and I was ready for it. A lot of bad first experiences probably happened because the girls weren't ready or the guy just wants to get laid and they're not considerate. I don't know; I had a good one.

My parents were split up and I was staying with my mom. I was visiting her for the summer. My father had a slight issue with it when he found out because the guy was 21 and I was 15 and he said, "No way in hell." And I said, "Well, it's already a done deal so... meet him and deal with it because you can't turn it back and fix it. So deal with it as a parent from that point on." He met the guy and didn't like him. But it all went well I guess you could say.

I had a great experience and it was because I was ready and I had a great guy who gave me a good time. And that's what you should wait for.

He eventually sort of became of the mindset that we were having some sort of relationship. Two weeks after it began he was like, "Oh, I ran into my ex-lover and I'm moving to San Francisco." I was like, "Dude, this meant nothing. You were practice."

Isaac, 41
Chicago, Illinois

LAURA'S STORY
Laura, 37

The first person to take my virginity, and I say the first person to take it because I choose to think of the first person as being the person that I loved and cared for. However, the first person to take my *physical* virginity was a nasty and horrible situation. I still look back and think that was really strong of me not to consider the horrible experience to be my loss of virginity.

At 15 I was pretty brutally raped. I was cut, beat up, everything. The choice was taken away from me. It wasn't until I was almost 19 that I chose to think I really lost my virginity, by my decision, with a person who was smart and attractive and I very much loved and who I dated for almost a year before we had sex.

He and I used to park, that was the big thing for us, and we would maul each other, do oral sex. The first act of intercourse happened on one of the cold, winter nights we were parked at a golf course, ironic because neither of us played golf. We had been talking about sex for months. I thought my own reticence to have sex was odd or unnatural but I learned that he, having not gone through anything violent, was just as reticent as I was. I feel he would have been equally hesitant had I not gone through something nasty, so that made it special. He didn't treat me like some mental patient. He knew about the rape and we both agreed wholeheartedly that that shouldn't mean anything. He was a virgin for real so the first time was really important for the both of us.

It was classic. This was in the dead of winter up in "Siber-acuse," upstate New York. We were in a dumb car with this stupid stick shift and as the moment approached we took a time-out and talked about it and we asked each other, "Is this OK?" We loved each other and it was tender and emotionally wonderful, while physically it was a little awkward and scary and frankly not very satisfying. As a woman it hurt. I think for a lot of teenage boys, sex is just masturbating into a woman. They don't understand that women have different equipment down there that needs to be serviced a little differently. It was cold out; I'm sure that made things difficult for him.

After the fact, I jumped out of the car to pee and I saw blood in the snow, which was a little confusing since physically I wasn't a virgin. But on an emotional level there was a relief like, "Wow. We finally did it." It wasn't kismet or anything but it was an important milestone in our relationship and it felt that our relationship had transgressed into something bigger.

Immediately after though, it was awkward and silly and stupid. It was a silent car ride home. Even the next morning when we called each other, we were really awkward toward each other and we had never been awkward with one another. And the truth of the matter was the reason we even had sex was because we were so comfortable with one another. The first time was so bad and fumbling that it turned into an inside joke between us. The first time is never *good* but it always gets better.

I think it's important to note that this is a person I did not go on to marry. There was no fairytale ending, but he remains a friend to this day. We still talk and send the occasional email.

My first time was sort of a dual experience. There was the person who I loved very much, and there was that person I didn't even know, that evil, nasty piece of work who put me in the emergency room and almost killed me. But I refuse to allow the bad rape situation as the defining moment.

(…and how not to)

CONCLUSION

If you picked up this book as a virgin looking for definitive steps as the best way to lose it, hopefully you were guided in the right direction. Ultimately, you yourself know the best way to lose it for you. As interviewer and editor, here is what I learned:

First, women like to talk about sex, just as much if not more so than men. So, if on the cusp of your first time and you have a partner picked out, you're both probably nervous. Thus, talking about it is a smart move. For one thing, it's good to be on the same page about how each of you feels regarding the possibility of sex, what you want out of it. You might even find that it's something your partner enjoys talking about.

It's important to be truthful with yourself and the other person about what you expect. If you are looking for love then it will most likely work best if your partner feels the same way. If you are just looking to get the first time over with than a partner who has the same attitude would most likely produce the best results. I have found through many of these stories that a shared outcome, an equality of desire, so to speak, makes for positive memories. One person wanting love while the other just wanting a lay leads to hurt feelings. Honesty is the best policy, and that holds true in the bedroom.

Granted, sometimes you will find yourself in a situation where a partner has been less than honest about their intentions in the bedroom (or even beyond), but perhaps they were unsure of what they wanted. There exist plenty of examples within these pages of first times that did not go as planned, felt wrong, or lacked the magic they were hoping for. We can't always choose where life takes us, but we can choose how we handle life , how we respond to these situations. It is possible to grow from a less than desirable first time into a sexually capable individual. If it was bad once, it does not have to be bad the rest of your life. Even some of the interviewees with traumatic loss of virginity stories, after time and support from loved ones, have grown from the past into a healthy present and future.

So how do you lose your virginity? It probably can be easily summed by quoting the Golden Rule, Aretha Franklin, and any number of Beatles songs...

Honesty, R-E-S-P-E-C-T, Love.

Be careful. And enjoy!

(...and how not to)

SPECIAL THANKS

Brooke Willis, Jenni Barker David Levin, Sarah Nowak for their keen eyes and proofreading skills.

Dad and Kathy for supporting the idea.

Melissa, Scott, and my nephew Ricky for keeping a spare room back in Cleveland.

Desireé Nash for believing and encouraging.

Joe Buccier who was my "wingman" during some early interviews before I had worked up the courage to go it alone.

Elana Fishbein for her support and affirmation along the way.

David Levin for driving (wasn't that fun?). Yang Miller for his unending generosity.

Jason Calicchia who had a lot of opinions about this book, most of which were right.

Lou Caravella for making this book one of his special projects.

Johnny Wu & Ray Elkin for being a pair.

Pat Shields for teaching men to fish.

Ryan Weyls for his scathing wit.

UCB, The PIT, the Magnet and everyone in the NY improv community without whom I'd have a very small support system.

Simple Studios rehearsal space – SimpleStudiosNYC.com

Diana DePasquale for very early proofreading.

Models: Lindsay Bane, Mike Capritta, Kathryn Dunn, Samantha Gurewitz, Amanda Harris, Lucas Zachary Hazlett, Nico Jordan, Abigail, Murphy, Crystal Powell, Roman Rimer, Rachel Werbel, Phil Wells

Photographers: Emily Bryan, Keith Huang

Designers: Jonathan Kaplan, Rick Koston (whose story resides somewhere within these pages)

All the helpful and friendly people at CreateSpace.

Made in the USA
Lexington, KY
12 April 2010